A TEXTBOOK OF PHARMACEUTICS I

AS PER LATEST PCI SYLLABUS FOR B.PHARM I YEAR STUDENTS

DR. SHIKHA BAGHEL CHAUHAN

Made with ♥ on the Notion Press Platform
www.notionpress.com

Contents

Preface

The Textbook of Pharmaceutics I for B.Pharm Semester I aims to develop the understanding of the formulation of a pure pharmacological component into a dosage form. This course is designed to impart a fundamental knowledge on the preparatory pharmacy with arts and science of preparing the different conventional dosage forms.The syllabus content is organised unit-by-unit in which each unit contains different chapters to promote better subject understanding.

Objectives: Upon completion of this book the student should be able to:

- Know the history of profession of pharmacy
- Understand the basics of different dosage forms, pharmaceutical incompatibilities and pharmaceutical calculations
- Understand the professional way of handling the prescription
- Preparation of various conventional dosage forms

This book features examples of formulation, including marketed goods and manufacturers, wherever necessary, along with full forms and symbols, pictorial diagrams, and tabular data. At the conclusion of each chapter, sample questions are provided for practise on the material covered in each chapter.

We are highly thankful to our students Palak Gupta, Gayatri Singh, Kishori Gupta, Shivam Pathak, Shweta Thakur, Reshna Renji, Anshika Rana, Rupali Verma and Neha Ghosh for their chapter contribution and their consistent effort and hardwork in the completion of the book.

Acknowledgements

It is our immense pleasure to publish and present this book of Introductory Pharmaceutics I (B.Pharm I Semester) to the pharmaceutical sciences students, teachers, and research scholars.

The authors are highly thankful to our students Palak Gupta , Gayatri Singh , Kishori Gupta , Shivam Pathak, Shweta Thakur , Reshna Renji , Anshika Rana , Rupali Verma , Neha Ghosh for their continous support and for their contribution of book chapters. We would never have been able, to complete this book without their support and motivation. We are highly thankful to **Dr. Sandeep Arora sir** (Director, Amity Institute of Pharmacy, Amity University, Noida) for always providing support, motivation, and constant encouragement. I hope this book will help the students in understanding the core concepts of subject and develop deep understanding of subject.

The readers of this book are requested to present their reviews and suggestions which will be highly appreciated and accepted by the authors. Constructive suggestions, comments and criticism on the subject matter of the book will be gratefully acknowledged, as they will certainly help to improve future editions of the book.Our special thanks to the publisher for bringing out the good quality printed book.

CHAPTER I

Historical Background and Development of Profession of Pharmacy

HISTORICAL BACKGROUND

INTRODUCTION

The word "pharmacy" derived from the Greek word "pharmakon," which meaning "drug." The use of medications in a safe and effective manner is the responsibility of the health profession, which connects the health sciences with the chemical sciences. Pharmacy is often described as a profession involved with the art and science of selecting appropriate medications from both natural and synthetic sources and administering them for medication diagnosis, prevention, and treatment.

ORIGIN OF PHARMACY

Around Baghdad in the ninth century, the pharmacy profession began to take shape in the developed world. Alchemy was used to gradually spread throughout Europe before becoming chemistry. The first known chemical method for making medication was carried out by artists in numerous nations including Asia, Mesopotamia, Egypt, and China. However, it entirely emerged from medicine and evolved as a new profession in the 19th century. The practise at the time was limited to manufacturing, mixing, and delivering medications in bulk numbers rather than for general sale. In contrast to the sophisticated pharmacological treatments of this age, medicine was solely administered through elixirs, spirits, and powders.

HISTORY OF PHARMACY

A long history of the pharmacy profession can be traced back to Samaria in the third millennium BC. On clay tablets, the Samarian people penned something akin to cuneiform writing that included lists of drugs with plant, animal, and mineral sources that were used to treat illnesses as well as prescriptions that included information on the ingredients needed to prepare them. The Greeks were one of the earliest ethnic groups to support the pharmacy industry. The Sumerians who previously lived in what is now Iraq are the originators of this field of study. The knowledge of how to prepare and use natural ingredients for healing is as old as man himself. The first written accounts of the production of medicines are from Babylonia, 2600 BC. They demanded a combination of healing, preventative, and spiritual measures. The Ebers Papyrus, which dates back to 1550 years.

These pharmacists were priests who served in the temples, just as the Sumerians. A field of medicine with significant prestige was considered to be pharmacy. A continuous scroll measuring 60 feet long and 1 foot wide, the Ebers Papyrus was composed around the year 1500 A.D. It has 800 prescriptions and 700 medicines (formulas). Most medicines are made from plants, such as acacia, castor bean, fennel, etc. Medications that the Egyptians produced and utilised include infusions, ointments, lozenges, suppositories, lotions, enemas, and pills, according to the literature. Milk, honey, beer, and wine served as the carriers. Many pharmaceutical formulations had twenty or more different types of medications. In China, a detailed concept of diagnosis and therapy was developed. The work Huangdi Nejing described the basics of employing pharmacological medications in the third century BC. Ayurvedic medicine was first documented in India around 800 BC. The god of medicine, Dhanvantari, and the use of charms and remedies to ward off demons are mentioned in documents. According to the "Charaka Samhita," drugs having plant, animal, and mineral origins were employed up to the first century AD. Hippocrates is recognised as the "Father of Medicine" (460 BC). He is connected to a number of books from the 420–370 BC era known as the Hippocratic Corpus, which lists 200–400 botanically derived medicines and instructs readers on how to prepare gargles, ointments, and pessaries.

King of Pontus (present-day Turkey), Mithridates (134–63 BC), experimented with poisons and antidotes, testing them on both captured foes and himself. Up until their crucifixion in 304 AD, Damian and Cosmas, two identical Arabian Christians, co-practiced medicine and pharmacy. Dioscorides, a Greek physician and botanist, is well known for his writings on botany as a subfield of pharmacy. He lived from 40 to 90 AD. Dioscorides composed De Materia Medica between the years 60 and 78 AD. Galen was a physician in the year 160 AD. He used the texts of Dioscorides and Hippocrates to compile the medical knowledge of the day. He talked about the usage of galenicals, or mixtures produced from various plants. In ancient Japan, pharmacists were held in great regard. In the Imperial family, the pharmacist even held a position of responsibility.

Monks who were trained as apothecaries preserved advanced knowledge during the Middle Ages (5 to 12 centuries), and they raised medicinal herbs in cloister gardens for the treatment of sick and injured people under their care. The Arabic period, which spans from the 7th to the 12th century, is regarded as the period of transmission of the cultural and scientific heritage of Antiquity and of the East to the West. The 9th century saw the development of the pharmacy profession in the civilised region surrounding Baghdad. It began as alchemy and gradually spread throughout Europe before becoming chemistry. The artists of Mesopotamia, Egypt, and China performed the first chemical reaction that is recorded in history.

During the Middle Ages (5 to 12 centuries), monks who had received apothecary training kept sophisticated knowledge and grew medicinal herbs in cloister gardens for the care of those who were ill or hurt. The cultural and scientific wealth of Antiquity and the East was transmitted to the West during the Arabic period, which runs from the 7th to the 12th century. In the affluent area surrounding Baghdad, the pharmacy profession began to emerge in the ninth century. Alchemy was the starting point, and as it expanded slowly across Europe, chemistry emerged. The earliest chemical reaction ever recorded in history was performed by artists in Mesopotamia, Egypt, and China.

Frederic II developed a constitution in 1231 that incorporated medical legal norms from the Arab world. He divided medicine into three categories: manual medicine, which performs surgical procedures, dogmatic medicine, which makes diagnoses, and pharmaceutical medicine, which collects, blends, and saves drugs. Pharmacy practise has existed for a long time. Pharmacists were frequently referred to as Sayadilah and Sandali in Arabic and Latin literature. The same Arabs who built pharmacies also expanded the supply of medicines. Mohammedans and Arabs crossed paths on their way to Mecca. This made it possible for people from India, China, and Spain to exchange goods and ideas, which sparked the development of various new medications in the medical field. Arabs have created cutting-edge medication delivery systems, such as syrups, pellets, and preserves.

Apothecaries were individuals who resided in London and had passed the examinations of the Worshipful Society of Apothecaries of London, established in 1617, between the years of 1600 and 1800. The job of the apothecary developed from that of the spicer, who manufactured pharmaceuticals and traded unprocessed drugs. Apothecaries handled chemicals and drugs, conducted medical examinations, and provided patient care in addition to their significant involvement in distributing. Apothecaries did not charge for these services; they only charged for the drugs they sold. Apothecaries were recognised as members of the medical profession who could suggest and dispense remedies in the Rose Case (1701-1703-4) ruling.

In the 19th century, pharmacy completely distanced itself from medicine and started to develop as a separate profession. This century saw the passing of many significant milestones in the field of pharmacy. In Philadelphia, Pennsylvania, doors of the country's first "School of Pharmacy" were first opened in 1821. the first U. S. Pharmacopoeia was published in 1820. The American Pharmacist Association was founded in 1852. The first "National Formulary" was published in 1888.

HISTORY OF PHARMACY IN INDIA

The development of the pharmacy profession in India can be split into three eras: pre-independence, independence, and post-independence.

Ancient Pharmacy Profession:

- In ancient India, the sources of drugs were of vegetable, animals and mineral sources, they were prepared by few experienced person and the knowledge of the medication was kept as a secret within the family.
- In mythology, it was assumed that Lord Brahma was the first teacher of the universe, who wrote "Ayurveda" in 500 B.C.
- The Ayurveda work on internal medicine, whereas Sushruta-Samhita deals mainly with the surgical medications. A book was also written ("Charaka Samhita") by Charaka and Sushruta who were physicians as well as pharmacists and studied more than 1000 herbs.

- After that, Egyptians and Greek scholars has contributed much in initial stages. The **Ebers Papyrus** (1550 BC) was the first who systematically discovered the classification of medicines.
- **Hippocrates** (400 BC) is referred as the father of medicines.
- The ancient Greek physician **Galen** (181-201 AD) reported methods of preparation of drugs from plants, which are called Galenicals.
- The first general hospital was set up at madras in the name of Madras Medical College in 1835, where professional training was given to students for treating patients with drugs.

Pre-Independence Pharmacy Profession:

- The beginning of this profession was started in 19th century, when the first chemist shop was opened by Scotch Bathgate at Calcutta in 1811.
- In 1840, Goa Medical college was started at Panjin. "Bengal Dispansatory" and Pharmacopeia was published in 1841 at Bishop`s College Press Calcutta and the order is given by the Government.
- In 1868, Pharmacopoeia of India was published under the editorship of warring.
- In 1878,`opium act' was implemented that deals with cultivation of poppy and manufacture, transport, export, import and sale of opium.
- In 1889, Indian Merchandise Act was implemented to avoid misbranding of gods. Health Scenario in India during 1901-1980 was not good. The people were under the poverty line and were undernourished and the systems of treatment for the prevention of diseases were under ayurvedic, allopathic and unani system of medicine

Post-Independence Pharmacy Profession:

- In 1948, Indian Pharmaceutical Congress Association (IPCA) was formed at Calcutta. IPCA is the apex body representing the Indian pharmacists working in various units in India.
- The Pharmacy Act was came in force in 1948, which provide statutory regulation for pharmacy institutions in india. Under this act, "the Pharmacy Council of India"(PCI) was established in 1949.
- First D.Pharma course was started in1949 at Institute of Pharmacy in West Bengal. The first "Education Regulation" was framed in 1953. In 1953, PCI made D.Pharma course as a compulsory minimum qualification ton work as a Pharmacist in India.
- The first edition of Indian Pharmacopoeia was published in 1955 and includes all the drugs formulations from variety of sources.

PHARMACY EDUCATION IN INDIA

Up to the beginning of the 19th century, India lacked a pharmacy education. Only conventionally experienced people were active in medicine, and there was no recognised or specialised schooling in this field. Pt. Madan Mohan Malaviya added "Pharmaceutical Chemistry" as a new subject to the three-year science bachelor's degree programme following the report's release (B.Sc.).

The first B.Pharm course at BHU was launched in 1937 by Mahadeo Lal Shroff, known as "The Father of Pharmacy Education in India." The first issue of Journal is India Indian Journal of Pharmacy was released in 1939. At BHU, the first post-graduation course was originally offered in 1940. The "Doctor of Philosophy" (Ph.D.) programme was established at BHU in 1945. The Drugs Act of 1940's Drugs Rule was enacted the same year.

To regulate pharmacy education in India, the Indian government introduced the pharmacy bill in 1945. Col. RN. Chopra served as the publication's chairman as The Pharmacopoeial List was released in 1946. The List includes medications used in India that were excluded from the British Pharmacopoeia. In 1947, the Legislature passed the "Pharmacy Bill" to oversee, regulate, and standardise pharmacy education in India.

Regulations for the Bachelor of Pharmacy (Practice), 2014

A two-year transitional programme to advance diploma holders into the bachelor's level was started by the Pharmacy Council of India through the 18 December release of the Bachelor of Pharmacy (Practice) Regulations, 2014. Students who earn a diploma in pharmacy (D. Pharm) will need to finish a two-year pharmacy bridging course before they can register with the State Pharmacy Councils as of 2017. As a result, in order to practise within two years, all new pharmacists will need to obtain a degree-level qualification. The goal is to modernise pharmacy credentials and standards to a uniform degree level across the country. This initiative will include patient counselling, hospital pharmacy administration, and community pharmacy management.

The 2014 Regulations for the Bachelor of Pharmacy (B. Pham.) and Master of Pharmacy (M. Pharm.)

The Pharmacy Council of India, with the Central Government's approval, published The Bachelor of Pharmacy (B.Pham) and Master of Pharmacy (M. Pharm.) Course Regulations, 2014 on December 10th. The duration of the course is specified by the new legislation. The minimum criterion for enrollment in this course is a B-level syllabus. The organisation and format of the tests, as well as the Pharm and M.Pharm courses In accordance with this law, PCI has implemented a choice-based credit system for pharmacy courses. The guiding principles of the Credit Based Semester System state that a particular quantity of academic work, i.e. The evaluation of things like theory classes, practical classes, and tutoring hours is done using credits. after passing the required courses.

The 2015 Pharmacy Practice Regulations

The Pharmacy Practice Regulations, 2015, are enacted by the Pharmacy Council of India on January 15, 2015, in accordance with the powers conferred by Sections 10 and 18 of the Pharmacy Act, 1948 (8 of 1948), and with the approval of the Central Government. Only licenced registered pharmacists are allowed to provide medications, under the regulations. Renting pharmacy owners registration certificates is utterly prohibited. During working hours, pharmacists are required to wear a white, spotless apron with a black badge plate bearing their name and registration number. The pharmacists whose registration certificates were rented out without their participating in dispensing services were deemed to have engaged in misconduct and had their registration certificates permanently revoked.

PHARMACEUTICAL INDUSTRY IN INDIA

Ayurveda, the Indian system of medicine, did not create its medications on an industrial scale prior to the year 900. For pharmaceutical products, India was heavily dependent on the UK, France, and Germany.

Acharya Prafulla Chandra Ray founded a tiny industry called the Bengal Chemical and Pharmaceutical Works in Calcutta in 1901. Prf. Tk. Gujjar founded the Alembic Chemical Works, a tiny industry in Mumbai, in 1903.

Hindustan Antibiotics Ltd., which was founded in Pune in the 1950s, is a major player in allopathic medications, particularly antibiotics. India's pharmaceutical sector has grown remarkably over the past few decades. The post-General Agreement on Tariffs and Trades era's enhanced reporting and technical development can be blamed for the rapid expansion.

The government did, however, use both native and foreign technologies to establish Hindustan Antibiotics Limited (HAL) and Indian Drugs and Pharmaceuticals Limited (IDPL) in the 1950s. This provided the necessary momentum and inspired some trust in the private industry participants during the last stages of the pharmaceutical sector's development. The business sector, which has significantly improved its reverse engineering capabilities, also appreciates the contribution made by the CSIR Laboratories. post 1970. The late 1960s and early 1970s saw a conscious effort to disseminate information.

The socialist platform of the government and a careful examination of rules and regulations that would restrict local engagement prepared the way for the growth of India's domestic generic sector. The Ayyangar report, which examined the law, said that foreign patent holders controlled the market due to a large number of approved patent applications. It was stated that the nation's interests were not served by the current patent laws. The Patents Act of 1970, which restricted patents for medicines and agricultural substances to just the processing stage, was Due to the early work of a select group of indigenous people, the modern pharmaceutical industry got off to a strong start. The British government established the Bengal Chemical and Pharmaceutical Works (BCPW), created in 1892, as one of the medical schools to provide training in current pharmaceutical research. It has also been noticed that other persons have made similar attempts in the past. In the 1930s, efforts were launched to make synthetic bulk pharmaceuticals with the aim of meeting around 13% of India's pharmaceutical product demand. Several additional domestic enterprises produced medications throughout and after World War II.

The penetration of medical facilities, occurrence of chronic diseases, increase in per capita income, and expansion of health insurance coverage are all factors that will contribute to the expansion of the domestic pharmaceutical market. The main global branded pharmaceuticals' patent expirations, notably in the US market, would be a significant factor boosting India's exports of pharmaceutical products. The expansion in the US market will be driven by rising generic formulations and a robust Abbreviated New Drug Application (ANDA) stream from Indian pharmaceutical companies. Developing nations like South Africa, Russia, Brazil, and others will aid in the long-term expansion of the export market, along with a stronger emphasis on specialised and challenging product categories.

PHARMACIST

A certified veterinarian, medical, or dental practitioner must write a written prescription in order for a pharmacist to be trained and licenced to formulate, combine, and dispense drugs. The scope of the pharmacy profession also includes more modern tasks including clinical services, evaluating medications for safety and efficacy, and providing drug information. Compounding and distributing pharmaceuticals are also included in this. Pharmacists work in the creation of drugs and other health-related items as well as in the management of the pharmaceutical businesses. Pharmacists, who are specialists in drug therapy, are the primary healthcare providers who maximise the use of medication for the benefit of patients.

PHARMACY AS A CAREER

A career in pharmacy is among the best jobs there are. Healthcare services include pharmacy, whose manufacturing and research have developed dramatically in recent years. Research, development, formulation, quality assurance, packaging, storage, marketing, and distribution are all covered by this area of pharmaceutical sciences, which has attained independent status. According to Dr. B. Suresh, the President of the Pharmacy Council of India, contrary to popular belief, the rise in hospitals, nursing homes, and pharmaceutical companies worldwide is a glaring indication of the expanding field of pharmacy, offering excellent and rewarding career opportunities in terms of jobs as well as the opportunity to launch one's own business.

SCOPE IN PHARMACY

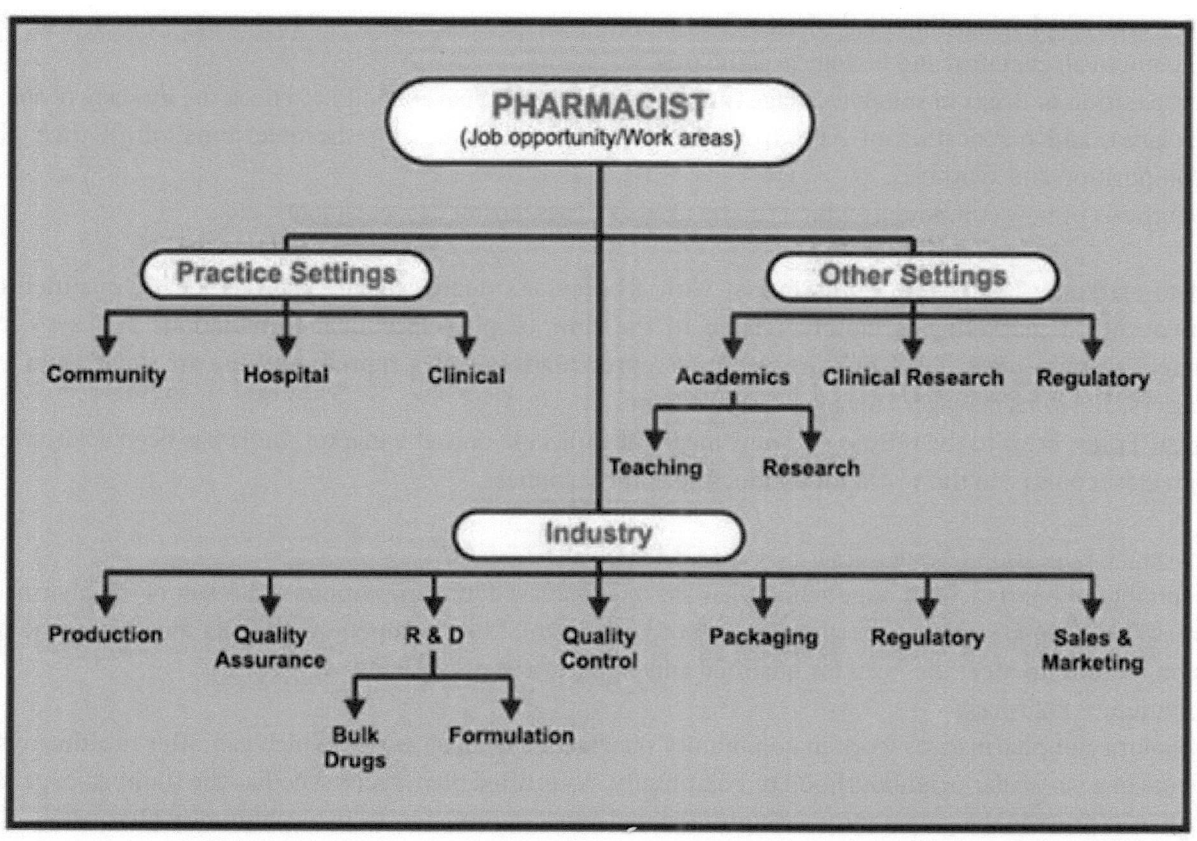

Scope of Pharmacy

The range of a pharmacy comprises a number of industries, including retail, medical facilities like hospitals and clinics, nursing homes, and pharmaceutical companies. In addition to roles like compounding and dispensing medications, modern services related to patient care now include clinical services, reviewing for safety and efficacy of the medications, and providing drug information. These areas of practise include hematology/oncology, infectious diseases, nutrition support, drug information, paediatrics, etc.

DIFFERENT PHARMACY PRACTICE AREAS

1.Wholesale Pharmacy

It gives a small number of pharmacists the chance to operate a wholesale pharmacy for drugs and medications. Between the manufacturer and the store, the wholesalers play an intermediary role.

2.Industrial Pharmacy

The pharmaceutical sector provides employment prospects for pharmacists in the following fields and at all educational levels:

- Production: A pharmacist with a bachelor's degree in pharmacy can operate as a manufacturing chemist in this industry. He is responsible for controlling the manufacturing, packaging, labelling, and storage of pharmaceutical formulations.
- Analytical and Quality Control: In this industry, manufacturing facilities require the services of analytical chemists for their analytical laboratories, where a pharmacist with a bachelor's in pharmacy can find employment as an analytical chemist to conduct testing on the raw materials and completed goods produced by the facility.
- Research and Development and New drug discovery : Most pharmaceutical companies in this field have their own independent research and development unit, where a pharmacist with a doctorate or master's degree in pharmacy is most suited. This department works in the following areas:
    - Research on pharmacokinetics, pharmacodynamics, pharmacovigiliance and toxicology of new drugs to study the physical, chemical and biological standards.
    - Preparation of drugs in suitable dosage forms and testing its bioavailability to check the efficacy of the drugs.
    - Isolation and purification of APIs from plant and animal tissues for the determination of their chemical composition and synthesis.
    - Synthesis of new compounds which can be used as drugs, cosmetics, excipients, etc.
- Medico-marketing and sales: A pharmacist with a bachelor's degree in pharmacy is ideally qualified because pharmaceutical marketing is closely related to the flow of pharmaceutical formulations and services from producer to customers. Field officers, medical representatives, sales representatives, area managers, regional managers, and sales managers make up the sale team.
- Clinical Trials: Prior to the release of a new medicine molecule onto the market, India has been acknowledged as the greatest country in the world for conducting clinical studies.

3.Pharmacy Education (Academics)

The number of pharmacy teaching schools has sharply increased in many nations as a result of the pharmaceutical companies' rapid expansion and the globalisation of health care. More competent students must enter the teaching profession in order to meet the need for qualified and experienced professors.

4.Community Pharmacy

The majority of pharmacists work in community pharmacies or drug stores, which can offer healthcare services to residents of a particular neighbourhood or community. A certified pharmacist who has the training, expertise, and competence to provide the community with professional services often works in a community pharmacy.

5.Hospital Pharmacy

Hospital pharmacists are professionals in the field of medications who work in hospitals, primarily in the public sector. They are in charge of purchasing, manufacturing, and quality testing all medications and drugs used in hospitals in addition to issuing prescriptions. Many hospital pharmacists are licenced to write the prescription for the drug.

6.Clinical Pharmacy

Clinical pharmacists offer a direct patient care service that optimises drug use, encourages good health, and works to ward off disease. Hospitals and clinics were where clinical pharmacists first started working in the clinical pharmacy. To enhance patient care, clinical pharmacists frequently work alongside doctors and other medical specialists.

7.Veterinary Pharmacy

Animal pharmacies, which are another name for veterinary pharmacies, can be found in both hospital and retail settings. To meet the medical needs of animals, veterinary pharmacies carry a variety of drugs.

PHARMACOPOEIA

The Greek terms "pharmakon" and "poleo," which mean "create" and "drug," respectively, are the source of the English phrase "pharmacopoeia." In the strictest sense, it alludes to a book that lists various drugs, raw medications, and recipes for creating preparations from them. The preparation of these books has been approved by the governments of the relevant countries. The books that list the requirements for medications and other related chemicals are referred to as "drug compendia."

These publications include a list of pharmaceuticals and other related chemicals together with details on their origin, descriptions, standards, tests, preparation formulae, actions and applications, doses, storage needs, and other information. Each new edition of these books includes some brand-new monographs, some that have been altered, and some that have been dropped. Industry leaders in the fields of medical, education, and pharmaceuticals wrote these books.

These pharmacopoeias, also known as national pharmacopoeias, are frequently developed with the consent of the government of the specific country.

National pharmacopoeias include, but are not limited to, the British Pharmacopoeia, the United States Pharmacopoeia, and others. The applicable pharmacopoeia covers the drugs or dosage forms that are currently most often used in that country because the medications utilised vary from country to country. The national pharmacopoeia will be cited when a dispute concerning pharmaceuticals arises since it is acknowledged as the reference book by the legislative authorities (by legislation) of the specific country.

IMPORTANCE OF PHARMACOPOEIA

- Pharmaceutical industry: When a new medication molecule is created, a considerable sum of money is spent on research and development. In poor nations like India, almost all medication firms are unable to cover the costs. In these circumstances, medications or other goods listed in pharmacopoeias may be marketed without further study. This is due to the tested, safe, and effective nature of the medications mentioned in pharmacopoeia. There are a number of standards in pharmacopoeia that raw materials used to make medicines and drugs must strictly adhere to. The pharmacopoeia is the most reliable source of knowledge about the accepted practises for drugs and pharmaceuticals, notwithstanding the existence of alternative sources. Since the authority has approved the assay techniques and identification tests for drugs and pharmaceuticals in pharmacopoeia, it is simple for business people to create the tests and employ the techniques with confidence.
- Drug-administration: Making money is every industry's primary goal. Some industries disregard the quality features of medications and pharmaceuticals as a result of this. Drugs affect both human and animal health, thus this carelessness is unacceptable. As a result, each country created its own drug-related Acts, Laws, and Rules. Pharmacopoeia is used as the first source of information regarding the product's quality in disputes between the government and the pharmaceutical industry.

- Academics: For information on how to utilise pharmaceuticals and drugs, consult the pharmacopoeias. Researchers always consult it directly when creating assay protocols for specific medications and assessing the efficacy of a dose form. The details on microbiological and bioassays are supplied as appendices. Consequently, the pharmacopoeia includes details on adverse effects, how to use pharmaceuticals and raw materials, and much more. The pharmacopoeia is favoured by students, academics, and educators due to the material's accuracy.

Classification

The drug compendia are classified as:

1.Official compendia: The government of the various nations of the origin of the drugs recognises official compendia as the collection of drugs and other associated substances that meet legal requirements of purity, quality, and strength. Among the official compendia are:

(a) British Pharmacopoeia.
(b) British Pharmaceutical Codex.
(c) Indian Pharmacopoeia.
(d) United State Pharmacopoeia.
(e) National Formulary.

2.Non-official compendia: Non-official drug compendia are those books that are utilised as secondary reference sources for drugs and other related substances in addition to official drug compendia. These consist of:

(a) Merck Index.
(b) Remington's Pharmaceutical Sciences.
(c) The United States Dispensary.

NATIONAL FOMULARY

The National Formulary of India (NFD) primarily acts as a reference for medical professionals that work in hospitals and retail settings, such as nurses, pharmacists, and medical students. This formulary was developed with the assistance of medical professionals, medical educators, nurses, pharmacists, and pharmaceutical manufacturers. The choice of which pharmaceuticals to include in the National Formulary was made after considering each drug's advantages and disadvantages, amount of utilisation in contemporary medical practise, and availability across the country. The NFI gives the doctor carefully selected therapeutic agents with proven efficacy and reflects a broad agreement of medical opinion regarding drugs and their formulations.

The IP's most recent version should be followed when selecting ingredients and formulas for the Formulary. Standards that were outlined in the IP edition prior to this one but weren't in the current edition would still be applicable. For drugs for which no standards have been established in the IP, the standards specified in the official pharmacopoeia of any other country where they are included shall apply. It's critical to abide by the Drugs and Cosmetics Act's regulations, particularly those pertaining to labelling and storage standards.

Indian Pharmacopoeia

By establishing authoritative and formally recognised standards for the quality of medications, including API, excipients, dosage forms, and medical devices used by healthcare professionals, patients, and consumers, the creation of IP was introduced with the goal of promoting public health.

The Indian Pharmacopoeial List, which the Indian government released in 1946, was used in addition to the British Pharmacopoeia. The Indian Pharmacopoeial List was prepared by a committee comprising nine other members and Sir R. N. Chopra as its chairman.

It was created in 1946 by the Government of India's Department of Health in Delhi. A committee to prepare the "Pharmacopoeia of India" was established by the Indian government in 1948, and its term was set at five years.

Under the leadership of Dr. B.N. Ghosh, the first edition of the Indian Pharmacopoeia Committee was produced in 1955. It is written in English with official monograph titles given in Latin. Under the direction of Dr. B. Mukherji, the Second Edition of IP was released in 1966, and official titles of monographs were given in English. After the medication monograph came the doses expressed in the metric system and the drug formulations.

The third edition of IP was released in 1985 and included 261 new monographs in two volumes and nine appendices. In 1989, Addendum I to IP was released, with 126 amendments and the addition of 46 additional monographs. When Addendum II was released in 1991, it contained 110 revised and 62 additional monographs.

Under the direction of Dr. Nityanand, the Fourth Edition of IP was published in 1996 and went into force on December 1st. It included 294 new monographs and 110 removed monographs, totaling 1149 monographs and 123 appendices. Addendum I, which includes 42 new monographs, became effective on December 31, 2000. Beginning on June 30, 2003, Addendum II went into effect, adding 19 more monographs.The veterinary addition to IP 1996, contains 208 monographs and four appendices.

The fifth edition of IP was released in 2007 and was distributed in three volumes, the first of which contains general notifications and chapters, the second and third of which contain general monographs on drug ingredients, dosage forms, and pharmaceutical aids.

The sixth edition of IP was released by the Indian Pharmacopoeia Commission (IPC), Ghaziabad, in 2010; it was available in three volumes and into effect on September 1, 2010. The Notices, Preface, Introduction, General Chapters, Acknowledgements, and IPC Structure are all found in Volume I. General Notice, General Monographs on Dosage Forms, and Monographs on Drug Substances, Dosage Forms, and Pharmaceutical Aids are all included in Volume II (A to M). Volume III includes monographs on medication ingredients, dosage forms, and medical devices (N to Z).

In this version, there are more monographs on vaccines, herbs and herbal products, blood and blood-related products, biotechnology products, and veterinary products. There are also more monographs on excipients, anticancer medications, herbal products, and antiretroviral pharmaceuticals.

The seventh edition of the Indian Pharmacopoeia, which was released in 2014 and presented in four volumes, was published by the Indian Pharmacopoeia Commission (IPC) on behalf of the Government of India's Ministry of Health and Family Welfare. It contains new anticancer medications and formulations, biotechnology products, native herbs and herbal products, and veterinary vaccines. Out of the 2550 drug monographs included in the IP 2014, 577 are brand-new monographs that include APIs, drug compounds, excipients, dosage forms, herbal items, etc.

British Pharmacopoela

The British Pharmacopoeia (BP) is an official set of standards for pharmaceuticals and medical devices in the UK. The BP, which is published yearly, includes monographs for pharmaceuticals, prepared medicines, and other pharmacological compounds used in medical practise.

Since 1864, the BP has provided authoritative, recognised standards for pharmaceutical ingredients and pharmaceutical products. It is still a crucial reference today and is used in approximately 100 different nations. It also includes fresh and updated monographs for mother tinctures, homoeopathic stocks, and herbal medicines.

The first edition of BP was released in 1864 and is divided into two parts: Part II: Preparation and Compounding and Part I: Materia Medica.

The next edition of BP was published in 1953, and in this edition, the names of medications and preparations were in English rather than Latin, and the units were in metric. The second edition of BP was published in 1867, followed by the third edition in 1884, the fourth edition in 1898, and the next edition in 1953.

BP 2007 saw the introduction of monographs for the ingredients needed to make traditional Chinese medicines.

With effect as of January 1, 2008, BP 2008 contains roughly 3100 monographs on drugs, preparations, and items used in practise.

Six volumes of BP 2007, 2008, and 2009 were distributed, and volumes I and II contain pharmaceuticals. Formulated preparations, immunological goods, radiopharmaceutical preparations, surgical supplies, and homoeopathic preparations are all included in Volume III. IR spectra are a set of supplemental chapters in Volume IV. Volume VI has a CD-ROM edition, and Volume V has veterinary.

BP 2010 contains 40 monographs for formed preparations, including veterinary pharmaceuticals and standards used for unlicensed formulations, and it becomes legally enforceable in the UK on January 1, 2010. Four volumes make up the set, together with one book of the BP (Veterinary) 2010.

The British Pharmacopoeia 2013 is divided into six volumes, including the BP (Veterinary) 2013, which includes 40 new European Pharmacopoeia monographs and 41 new BP monographs in addition to 619 amended monographs. then 619 revised monographs, including 6 new and 1 revised Infrared Reference Spectra, were published.

The only official source for British pharmaceutical standards is The British Pharmacopoeia 2014 The Human Medicines Regulations of 2012, which are produced and updated annually by the British Pharmacopoeia Commission Secretariat of the Medicines and Healthcare Products Regulatory Agency (MHRA), contain around 3500 monographs.

It has five volumes, including one volume of the BP (Veterinary) 2014, a fully searchable CD-ROM, and online access. It became legally binding on January 1, 2014, and it contained 272 modified monographs as well as 40 new BP monographs. Along with four new BP (Vet) monographs and one new BP (Vet) Supplementary Chapter, there were also three new Supplementary Chapters.

United State Pharmacopoeia

The United States Pharmacopoeia and National Formulary (USP-NF) is the official body in charge of establishing public standards for all prescription and over-the-counter medications as well as other healthcare items made or marketed in the country. Additionally, it had acknowledged standards for food ingredients and dietary supplements, which guarantee the quality, purity, potency, and consistency of goods produced for general use and are applied in more than 130 nations worldwide.

Volunteers from academics, government, the pharmaceutical and food businesses, health insurance, consumer organisations, and other health care professions participate in and oversee the programme.

The United States Pharmacopoeial Convention originally published the USP in 1820, and the American Pharmaceutical Association directed the publication of the National Formulary in 1888.

A book of public standards, the United States Pharmacopoeia-National Formulary (USP-NF) 2009, contains standards for drugs, dosage forms, drug substances, excipients, and nutritional supplements. It is offered in print, online, and CD media and is available in English.

The USP-NF is a three volume combination of two official compendia, the United States Pharmacopoeia (USP) and the National Formulary (NF). In the USP, monographs for drug substances and preparations are provided, and in the NF, excipient monographs are included.

Extra Pharmacopoeia

The Extra Pharmacopoeia, still referred to as "Martindale," was first published in 1883 by William Martindale. It is a recognised reference work on medications that is used globally. It provides the most recent information on medications such as selected,investigative, and veterinary drugs, herbal and complementary medicines, pharmaceutical excipients, vitamins, and nutritional agents, vaccines, radiopharmaceuticals, contrast media, and diagnostic agents.

The twenty-eighth edition was released in December 1982, followed by the twenty-ninth edition in January 1989, both of which were published at the direction of the council of "The Royal Pharmaceutical Society of Great Britain and prepared in the Society's Department of Pharmaceutical Sciences."

QUESTIONS

Q1. Describe the history and advancement of the pharmacy profession in India.

Q2. Describe the development of Indian pharmaceutical education.

Q3. Describe the various professions available following pharmacy.

Q4. Write a note on the United States, British, and Indian Pharmacopoeias.

Q5. Make a brief note about:

- Indian National Formulary
- Extra Pharmacopoeia

CHAPTER II

Dosage Forms Introduction to dosage forms classification and definitions

PHARMACEUTICAL DOSAGE FORMS

DRUG

A substance referred to as a "drug" is one that is used to diagnose, mitigate, treat, cure, or prevent disease in humans or animals. Experts qualified by scientific training and experience to evaluate the safety and effectiveness of drugs refer to any drug whose composition is such that it is not generally acknowledged as safe and effective for use under the conditions prescribed, recommended, or suggested in the labelling of the drug as a "new drug."

SOURCES OF DOSAGE FORMS

Laxatives and anti-emetics were the most frequently used medications in the Middle East and China, where records of drug use date back to 2,700 BC. The drugs used to treat illnesses came from natural sources up until the final decade of the 19th century. Minerals, plants, and animals are examples of natural sources. Plants were primarily utilised among the natural sources. Animals and minerals have both been utilised for the same purpose on occasion. A considerable number of pharmaceuticals are derived from microorganisms today, while the majority of drugs are synthetic and made in laboratories. The following categories apply to drug sources:

PLANTS

Since ancient times, plants have been utilised to cure liver disorders with leaves that resemble the organ. Different plant parts, including the root, bark, stem, leaf, seed, and flower, are also employed as medicines. A certain medication is not equally present in all regions of a given plant. With a few exceptions, plants are no longer employed as medications in modern medicine; instead, pharmacologically active components (PAC) are isolated from plants and used instead. Alkaloids, glycosides, oils, gums, mucilage carbohydrates, and other related substances are all included in a plant's PAC. By soaking the plant in appropriate solvents, such as ether or alcohol, some of these active ingredients can be extracted.

ANIMALS

To alleviate toothaches and gum bleeding, the Chinese utilised dried toad skin that contains adrenaline. Omega-3 fatty acids, vitamin A, and vitamin D are present in high concentrations in cod liver oil, which is obtained from cod fish. Bovine or porcine pancreas are used to extract insulin. Antigen is injected into an animal to create immunoglobulin G, which is then made by removing the antibody produced in response to the antigen. To cure illnesses like measles, mumps, hepatitis, etc., human immunoglobulin is created from pools of at least 1000 human plasma donors. The preparation of hepatitis B immunoglobulin, rabies immunoglobulin, and tetanus immunoglobulins involves pooling the plasma from particular donors who have high concentrations of the necessary antibodies.

MINERALS

Iron was a common treatment for anaemia and weakness in ancient Greek medicine. Diarrhea has been treated with various clays, kadin, and activated charcoal. Calomel is used to treat congestive heart failure, syphilis, and constipation. It also has a diuretic effect. The treatment of goitre involves the use of iodine. In order to treat arthritis, gold is employed. Skin conditions are treated externally with sulphur. Magnesium trisilcate and aluminium hydroxide are both commonly used antacids. Magnesium sulphide is used to treat ecliptic seizures and reduce constipation.

The safest and most efficient way to administer medication to the body is through dosage forms. Dosage forms are essentially pharmaceutical products that are sold for usage and often contain both excipients and active medicinal ingredients.

LABORATORY RESOURCES

Most medications nowadays are made by chemically reacting two or more substances or components. When compared to pharmaceuticals obtained from plants or animals, laboratory-produced medications are safer, higher-quality, less expensive, and more potent. The majority of the analgesics, chemotherapeutic medicines, hypnotics, and local anaesthetics that are currently utilised are created in laboratories. Digoxin and salicylates, sulfonamides, apomorphine, homatropin human insulin, etc. are a few examples of these types of medications. Actinomycin, amphotericin, chloramphenicol, erythromycin, kanamycin, neomyci gentamicin, streptomycin, and tetracycline are antibiotics produced by the microorganism actinomycetes. Penicillin, griseofulvin, and cephalosporin are among the antibiotics made by the aspergillate group of fungi. Bacitracin and polymyxin B are antibiotics produced by the genus Bocil of bacteria.

NEED FOR DOSAGE FORM

1.To make medicine administration easier and to improve patient care compliance.

2. To improve the stability of medicines under standard storage settings.

3. To improve therapy's production, distribution, and effectiveness

4. Upon oral delivery, to shield the medication from stomach acid, enteric-coated tablets, as an illustration.

5. To mask a pharmacological substance's unpleasant flavours or odours, for example, flavoured syrups, coated tablets, and capsules are a few examples.

6. To enable the drug's inhalational effect.

PHYSICAL STATE

SOLID	Powder, tablet capsule caplet, cachet pill, lozenge cache capsule insufflation, dentifrice, effervescent granules, suppository etc
SEMI-SOLID	Gel, ointment, cream, jelly, paste etc
LIQUID	Solution, emulsion syrup elixir, magma, suspension, aromatic water, collodion, draught ear drop, eye drop nasal drop, mixture, enema, gargle, gel injection, irrigation liniment, lotion mouth wash spirit, spray, syrup, tincture, paint
GASEOUS	Aerosol spray, inhalation

ROUTE OF ADMINISTRATION

ORAL	Powder, tablet, capsule solution, emulsion, syrup, magma gel, cachet, pill.
PARENTAL	Solution, suspension, emulsion, tablet, implant.
TOPICAL	Ointment, cream, powder, paste, lotion, plaster, liniment ge transdermal patch.
URETHRAL	Suppository, douche, intrauterine device, pessary, vaginal ring tablet.
SUBLINGUAL	Lozenge, tablet.
OPHTHALMIC	Eye drop, ophthalmic gel, ophthalmic ointment, solution
INTRANASAL	Solution, spray, inhaler.
OTIC	Ear drop (solution or suspension).
RECTAL	Suppository, enema.

SITE OF ACTION

1. Skin: Lotions, creams, liniments, and ointments.
2. Eye - lotions, ointments, and solutions.
3. Tooth: Toothpaste and tooth powder.
4. Hand-washing products, creams, and lotions.
5.Foot: Creams, ointments, and powders for dusting.
6. Hair: Shampoos, conditioners, hair creams, and hair mending.
7. Nasal: Sprays, solutions, and inhalation

Solid dosage form

1. Unit dosage

- Tables
    - Lozenges
    - Buccal
    - Sublingual
    - Chewtable
    - Soluble
- Pills
- Cachets
    - Dry seal
    - Wet seal
- Capsules
    - Hard gelatin
    - Soft gelatin
- Powders
- Suppositories
    - Ear cones
    - Rectal
    - Vaginal
    - Nasal

2). Bulk Dosage Form

- Internal use
    - Fine powders
    - Granules
- External use
    - Ear powder
    - Snuff powder
    - Dusting powder
    - Tooth powder

LIQUID DOSAGE FORM

1. Monophasic

1) Monophasic
   - Internal use
     - Aqueous
       - Drops
       - Mixture
       - Solution
       - syrups
     - Hydroalcoholic
       - Elixirs
   - Oral use
     - Mouth wash
     - Gargles
     - Throat paints
   - Body cavity
     - Ear drops
     - Nasal drops
     - Douches
     - Enemas
     - Sprays
   - Tropical
     - Lotion
     - Solution
     - Liniments

2. Biphasic

   - Emulsion
     - Parental
     - Oral
     - Ophthalmic
     - external
   - Suspension
     - Parental
     - Oral
     - External
     - Ophthalmic

3).SEMI-SOLID DOSAGE FORM

- External use
  - Ointment
    - Oleagenous base
    - Absorption base
    - Water washable base
    - Emulsion
  - Paints
  - suppositories
- Internal use
  - Gels
  - Jellies

1. Aromatic water: They are saturated aqueous solution of volatile oils or volatile substances and used as flavouring agent. e.g. Camphor water.

Mainly used as flavouring agent.

2. Cachets: They are solid dosage form which are used for oral administration of nauseous and disagreeable drug substances.

3. Tinctures: Tinctures are a type of oral preparation that is sweet and viscous and contains medicine that is demulcent, sedative, or expectorant in nature.

4. Spirits: Spirits are an alcoholic mixture of volatile oils that are ingested for therapeutic purposes as well as for flavouring. Spirit can be applied externally while being inhaled. for instance, aromatic spirit of ammonia

5. Proof spirits are defined as a blend of alcohol and water that has one-twelfth as much water as alcohol.

6. Elixirs are intense, nauseating oral alcoholic preparations that are clean, liquid, flavor-infused, and frequently appealing in colour. EG. Benzaldehyde elixir, chloral hydrate, etc.

7. Syrups: Syrups are concentrated aqueous preparations that often comprise sugar or other comparable ingredients, with or without flavourings and pharmaceuticals. Sucrose is a 66.7% w/w solution in syrup IP.

8. Droughts: Droughts are oral liquid medications intended to be taken as a unit dose.

9. Drops: Drops are oral liquid preparations of powerful medications or vitamins that are administered directly.

10. Ear drops: These are liquid preparations for the ears that often contain the medicine suspended or dissolved in an appropriate solvent, such as glycerol or alcohol.

11. Eye drops comprise buffers, antioxidants, stabilisers, and preservatives and are aqueous and oily solutions or suspensions of one or more APIs intended for the eye sac.

12. Ointments: Ointments are semisolid preparations used in tropical settings, as on the skin or some mucous membranes. They often consist of fats, oils, and waxes of animal, vegetable, or mineral origin and are solutions or dispersions of one or more medications in non-aqueous bases.

13. Gargles: Gargles are aqueous solutions that are typically sold in concentrated form with instructions to dilute with warm water, such as phenol gargle, etc. Gargles are used to cure or prevent infections.

14. Creams: Creams are viscous semisolid forms that are typically pseudoplastic in character, without emulsions (for aqueous creams) or with emulsions (for oily creams). It consists of a number of phases, including crystalline substance made from fatty alcohol, distributed oil, free water, and viscoelastic gel containing fixed water.

15. Gels: Gels are transparent or translucent semisolid preparations that are made up of substances that have a gel-like consistency and are a solution of one or more active ingredients in appropriate hydrophilic or hydrophobic bases.

Pastes are semi-solid preparations for topical administration that are stiffer than ointments and used as absorbents. They differ from similar products in that they contain higher proportions of finely divided medications.

17. Tablets: These solid dosage forms are designed to be taken by mouth and are made either through compression or moulding techniques.

18. Capsules: Capsules are solid dosage forms that typically include one dose of medication sealed within a tiny, water-soluble shell that is constructed of gelatin, a water-plasticizer, and preservatives for the cap and body.

19. Pills: For oral administration, pills are round, tiny solid dose forms containing one or more active components. The most popular oral dose form in the past was a pill, but compressed tablets and capsules have mostly taken their place.

Phenolphthalein tablets, for instance.

20. Paints are solutions or dispersions of one or more active substances that are meant to be applied to the skin or mucosa of the mouth and throat, typically with the aid of a soft brush or cotton swab. A volatile solvent, like alcohol, is frequently used in skin paints. Alcohol soon evaporates, leaving a dry, film-like material that is of medicinal use. For instance, crystal violet paint.

21. Liniments are liquid or semi-liquid solutions that are applied to healthy skin and then rubbed into the afflicted area. They could be alcoholic, greasy, soapy, or emulsified solutions. The oily or soapy liniments are softer in action but more helpful when massage is necessary. Alcoholic liniments are typically employed for their rubefacient, counterirritant, moderately astringent, and penetrating actions. Never apply liniments to skin that is damaged or injured in any way. A camphor liniment, for instance.

22. Lotions are liquid or semi-liquid formulations designed to be applied to intact skin without rubbing. They typically comprise antiseptic, astringent, anaesthetics, germicides, protectives, or screening agents for prevention or treatment of various skin illnesses. They are either dabbed on the skin or put over an appropriate dressing and covered with water resistant material to inhibit evaporation. Calamine lotion, for instance.

23. Lozenges are solid dosage forms that contain medication in a base that has been sweetened and flavour added with the intention of dissolving gradually in the mouth. A firm sugar candy, glycerinated gelatins, or a mixture of sugar and enough gum to give it form may serve as the base.

24. Mouthwashes: Mouthwashes are aqueous solutions with one or more active ingredients that are intended to be used in contact with the mucous membrane of the oral cavity, typically after dilution with warm water. They may contain additives like alcohol, glycerine, artificial sweeteners, surfactants, flavouring, and colouring agents.

25. Nasal drops are solutions, suspensions, or emulsions having active chemicals that are meant to be injected into the nostrils, typically with the aid of a dropper. Although oily drops are uncommon, they are typically based on aqueous vehicles.

SOLID DOSAGE FORM

Powders make up the majority of solid dose forms, and they are typically treated to some extent to change their form.

Advantages:

1. Compared to liquids, solid drugs are more stable and have a longer shelf life. 2. Less shelf space is needed, and it is simple to package, handle, ship, and move.

3. Preservatives are typically not necessary unless the product contains unstable medications.

4. Since the medication is already in a unit measure, a precise single dose can be administered.

5. suitable for regulating drug distribution to get desired results.

6. Self-administration of solid drugs by patients is simpler.

Disadvantages:

1. The preparation of solid dosage forms is challenging and expensive. machines.

2. Children, those with acute illnesses, and elderly patients have trouble ingesting solid dosage forms.

3. Due to their ability to resist flow and compacting into dense structures, several medicines Low density and an amorphous nature.

4. Solid drugs are not an appropriate choice for people who are unconscious or
possess breathing tubes for the nose and mouth.

5. Solid drugs require more time to be dissolved, absorbed, and dispersed in the body.

6. For therapies that require instant effect, solid drugs are not fast enough.

POWDERS

Drug dosage forms intended for internal or exterior usage include powders. Bulk powder and split powder are the two categories for the powder. Divided powders are single-dose presentations of powder that are meant to be given to the patient as such, to be consumed in or with water. Bulk powders are described as powders that must be measured out by the patient as a dose and are supplied in large quantities in a container. Dusting powders are those used for the outside, whilst oral powders are meant for internal use. Fine medicinal (bulk) powders called "dusting powders" are meant to be applied to the skin using sifter-top containers.

(1) Bulk powder for internal use, such as the combinations of sodium chloride and dextrose and rhubarb.

(ii) External bulk powders such as tooth powder and talc dusting powder.

(iii) Medical dusting powders, such as Neosporin Powder and Canesten Powder; Zinc and Salicylic Acid Dusting Powder; Zinc, Starch, and Talc Dusting Powder; etc.

Advantages:

1. The easiest and most adaptable form to deliver and compound is powder.
2. In particular for children and newborns, it gives doctors the flexibility to adjust the standard medicine dose to the patient's needs.
3. Powders are reliable and difficult to react with when they are solid.
4. The powder's small particle size facilitates quick medication absorption.
5. Compared to liquid dose form, they are less incompatible.

Disadvantages:

1. Compounding powders requires considerable time.
2. The dosage of a medicine may be incorrect when given as powder.
3. Powders are more expensive because of individual dose packaging.
4. Instable powders have volatile, hygroscopic, oxidising, and deliquescent characteristics.
5. Dosages for powders can be off.
6. If instructions are not given clearly, the patient could not grasp the proper manner of use. For instance, the proper way to administer medication, how to make a powder solution, etc.
7. If the drug has a bitter or unpleasant taste, it is not suited for oral delivery.

GRANULES

Wet, dried, and ground into coarse pieces, granules are made of drug-containing powders. These are dry, free-flowing conglomerates with a diameter of 1 to 5 mm. The mixture is then pushed through a filter to achieve the desired granule size and dried. Compared to powders, granules are larger and typically more stable. Granules may be dissolved in water before to ingestion or may be placed on the tongue and swallowed with water. Examples include the stimulating laxative Senokot Granules .

Advantages:

1. Granulation could prevent the segregation of the powder mixture's components.
2. Granules are less likely to clump together and more resistant to humidity and the environment.
3. Compared to light and fluffy powders, they are more easily wetted by liquids and are more is preferred for dry goods that are meant to be dissolved or suspended.
4. Compared to powders, granules are easier to flow. When providing medicinal components from the hopper or feeding container into the tableting presses, the easy flow characteristics are crucial.
5. Granules can also reduce or remove dust.

Disadvantages:

1. Making granules is time consuming and its packaging is difficult.
2. They are bulky to carry about.
3. Powder particles may spill when they are being opened.
4. Sometimes granules cannot be processed to tablet or capsule and are to be formulated as suspension.

5. Drugs with an unpleasant taste cannot be formulated as granules and need to be filled in a hard capsule.
6. Volatile deliquescent, hygroscopic or oxygen-sensitive drugs are difficult formulate as granules.

TABLETS

Tablets are characterised as solid pharmaceutical dosage forms that can be compressed or moulded and contain active pharmacological ingredients with or without appropriate excipients.

Examples are Crocin (paracetamol) Tablets and Analgin Tablets (aspirin).

Advantages:

1. Tablets have a sophisticated appearance and are easy to consume.
2. They are straightforward, affordable, and prolong the stability of the medicine.
3. The easiest form to package, pack, and move
4. The tablet surface can be printed with the product identification mark.
5. There are numerous tablet models available, each with a different set of features
6. Tablets may contain many medications for synergistic effects.
7. Sugar coating can hide unpleasant tastes while improving patient acceptance.
8. Tablets deliver an exact dose without the need for dose measurement.

Disadvantages:

1. Tablet ingestion is challenging for both children and elderly people.
2. To identify good compatibility between the medicine and excipients in a tablet, numerous tests are necessary
3. Drug absorption from tablets varies amongst patients.
4. Low density and highly amorphous materials are exceedingly challenging to compress.
5. Drugs with slow dissolving or poor wetting cannot be made as tablets.
6. A tablet's delayed disintegration and digestion may cause irritation of the GI mucosa and bioavailability issues.

Types of Tablets:

(i) Tablets ingested orally:

1. Compressed tablet.

For example, Crocin Tablet (paracetamol).

2. Multiple compressed tablet.

For example, Mucinex Tablet (guaifenesin).

3. Repeat action tablet.

For example, Trital Tablet (phenylephrine, ascorbic acid, paracetamol).

4.Delayed release tablet.

For example, Enteric coated Bisacodyl Tablet.

5. Sugar coated tablet.

For example, Becovit® Tablet (multivitamin and minerals).

6. Film coated tablet.

For example, Flagyl Tablet (metronidazole).

7. Chewable tablet.

For example, Gelusil Tablet (alumina, magnesium and simethicone).

(ii) Tablets used in oral cavity:

1. Buccal Tablet.

For example, Oravig® Tablet (miconazole).

2. Sublingual Tablet.

For example, Vicks® Tablet (menthol).

3. Troches or Lozenges.

For example, Difflam® plus Tablet (lignocaine).

4. Dental Cone.

For example, Parasorb Cone (gentamicin).

(iii) Tablet ingested from other route

1. Implantation tablet.

For example, Nexplanon® Tablet (etonogestrel).

2. Vaginal tablet.

For example, Canesten Tablet (clotrimazole).

(iv) Tablets used to prepare solution:

1. Effervescent tablet.

For example, Dispirin® Tablet (aspirin).

2.Dispensing tablet.

For example, Enzyme Tablet (digiplex).

3. Hypodermic tablet.

For example, Morphine Sulphate Tablet

4. Tablet triturates.

For example, Enzyme Tablet (digiplex).

PILLS

Pills are spherical dosage forms created by consistently blending drugs with excipients such as binders, disintegrators, and other suitable diluents. Capsules and tablets have now almost entirely replaced pills. The term "Vati" refers to pills, which are widely used in ayurvedic medicine as a dosage form. Today, "pills" refer to any directly ingestible oral dose form, including tablets, capsules, and variations like caplets. Some medications are made to have sensory and communication components that, after being ingested, capture and wirelessly communicate physiological data.

Examples include Viagra, Kamagra, Detox®, Choice, and Unwanted 72 pills.

LOZENGES

Lozenges are a type of solid dosage form for medications with a sweetening, flavouring, and strong binding agent designed for gradual disintegration in the mouth.

By compression They may contain active substances intended for systemic absorption after ingesting but are typically used to treat localised mouth or throat infections or discomfort. Lozenges are the tablets created by the fusion or candy moulding technique.

Examples include lozenges containing compound bismuth, liquorice, nystatin, or clotrimazole.

PASTILLES

Pastilles are another name for moulded lozenges. Lozenges are harder than pastilles. The medication is made into a pastille with gelatin and glycerin for gradual disintegration in the mouth.

Examples are Rescue Pastille and Vocalzone Throat Pastille. TROCHES

Advantages:

1. Both paediatric and elderly patients can easily be given lozenges.
2. Its flavour is pleasant, and it prolongs the time that it is in touch with the oral cavity.
3. With the least number of tools and preparation time, pharmacists can make it on the spot.
4. Formulas can be patient-specific and are simple to modify.
5. Historically, lozenges have been employed for localised effects.

Disadvantages:

1. Children could mistakenly use it as candy.
2. Hand-rolled lozenges take skill and proper technique to prepare and create.
3. The majority of hand-rolled lozenges lack a classy aesthetic.
4. Making lozenges via moulding typically requires specialised moulds.
5. To produce good preparations, handling basic materials takes a specific combination of knowledge, expertise, and tenderness.

DENTAL CONES

Dental cones are tablet-based medications that are meant to be inserted into the empty socket after a tooth extraction. Dental cones' primary function is to stop the spread of harmful microorganisms linked to tooth extractions or to lessen bleeding. The main reason for using this tablet is to either reduce bleeding by using an astringent or coagulant-containing tablet or to inhibit the growth of bacteria in the socket by using a slow-releasing antibacterial component. Antibiotics and antiseptics might be present in the cones. It is designed to gently disintegrate or erode during a 20–40 minute period in the presence of a small volume of serum or fluid.

Example: Parasorb Dental Cone (gentamicin).

PESSARIES

Pessaries are solid unit dose forms of medication that can be moulded with the aid of a foundation or compressed into an appropriate shape for introduction into the vagina. There are three forms of pessaries: moulded pessaries, compressed pessaries, and vaginal capsules. Molded pessaries are cone-shaped and created similarly to moulded suppositories. Compressed pessaries come in a range of shapes and are made similarly to oral tablets through compression. The only physical differences between vaginal capsules and soft gelatin oral capsules are size and form. the other word for vaginal medication distribution. pharmaceuticals must be administered via the urethra and rectum. A therapeutic pessary is a medical device that resembles a diaphragm's outer ring.

Advantages:

1. Some medications must be taken as prescribed in order to reach adequate body concentrations.
2. When used as directed, there are no adverse effects on the entire body.
3. can have an impact on the rectal mucosa locally.
4. used to encourage bowel evacuation.
5. Avoid causing your stomach any discomfort.
6. Patients who are unconscious can use this (for example, during fitting).
7. can be used to prevent first-pass metabolism and allow medications to be absorbed systemically. 8. when elderly or young patients are unable to swallow oral medications.

Disadvantage

1.The acceptability of patients is a concern for pessaries.
2. Patients who are diarrhoea patients should not use it.
3. Sometimes the whole dosage of the medication used will be either too grating or ineffective higher quantity.
4. Because suppository typically encourages partial absorption, removal of the bowel.
5. Primary vaginitis, active pelvic inflammatory disease, latex allergy, a noncompliant patient, and a lack of certain follow-up are all contraindications to pessary insertion.

CAPSULES

A "capsule" is a solid unit dosage form of medication that contains one or more pharmaceuticals inside of a gelatin-based, essentially tasteless, hard or soft dissolving container.

(a) Capsules made of hard gelatin

Two cylindrical pieces make form a hard gelatin capsule: the cap, which is slightly bigger in diameter but shorter in length, and the base, which is slightly smaller in diameter but longer in length.

Ampicillin capsule and multivitamin capsule are two examples.

Advantages

1. They're smooth and slippery, making swallowing them simple.
2. suitable for compounds with a foul smell and bitter taste.
3. They come in a variety of colours, are affordable, and are appealing.
4. It needs minimum excipients
5. The material can be compacted with little pressure.

Disadvantages

1. For extremely soluble compounds like potassium chloride, potassium bromide, ammonium chloride, etc., this is not the right choice.
2. Highly efflorescent or deliquescent materials are not recommended
3. requires unique storage circumstances.
4. The first pass effects of medications given in capsules are shown in the liver.

(b) Capsules made of soft gelatin

Another name for capsules is "pearls." To contain solids, soft gelatin capsules are utilised. Soft gelatin capsules come in a variety of shapes, including tubes, spheres, and ovoids.

Advantages:

1. They release their contents fast and are simple to swallow.
2. They can cover up offensive tastes and odours.
3. They appear to be elegant.
4. Easily dissolve in the digestive system's gastric juices (GIT).
5. They might make the active component more bioavailable.
6. Chewable, extended-release, captabs, and other forms of gelatin capsules are available.
7. They can be used for ophthalmic preparations, such as Aplicaps and recta/vaginal suppositories.
8. These capsules have precise, accurate, and equal dosing.
9. They offer protection against fakes and are tamper-resistant.
10. Offer defence against oxidation, light, and deterioration.

Disadvantages:

1. It is challenging to include water-soluble components in capsules.
2. They are extremely sensitive to wetness.
3. Because of leaching and softening, efflorescent substance cannot be included.
4. Materials that deliquesce cannot be used because they might cause hardness. 5. They are generally more expensive than liquid dose forms and soft capsules.
6. Due to the fact that gelatin is usually derived from bone, they must follow particular dietary restrictions and pig and cow skins.

DELAYED-RELEASED CAPSULES

Enteric coated capsules with the goal of delaying the release of medication until the capsule has passed through the stomach are referred to as "delayed-release" capsules. When a delay is necessary to prevent issues with drug inactivation or gastric mucosal irritation, delayed-release capsules or, more frequently, encapsulated granules may be coated to resist releasing the drug in the gastric fluid of the stomach.

Examples include Nexium® DR Capsule and Omeprazole DR Capsule (esomeprazole).

EXTENDED-RELEASED CAPSULES

Extended-release capsules are designed in a way that makes the medication they contain available for a long time after intake. Such dosage formulations have also been referred to as "prolonged-action," "repeat-action," and "sustained-release."

Examples are morphine sulphate ER capsules and indomethacin ER capsules.

CAPLETS

A mix between a capsule and a tablet, a caplet is an oblong tablet. The capiet is just a tablet that has been coated or fashioned to resemble a capsule. The interior of a capsule is often made of powder or granular substance, whereas the interior of a caplet is solid. A caplet has the benefit of being simpler to swallow, more stable, and having a longer shelf life than a capsule.

Relafine Caplet (nabumetone), Ceptin Caplet (cefuroxime), and Renovit® Caplet are a few examples.

INSUFFLATIONS

An insufflator will blow or deeply inhale a medication that has been well mixed with dusting powder into body cavities like the ears, nose, tooth sockets, and vagina. The insufflations are used to either achieve a systemic effect from a drug that is degraded in the GIT or to provide a local effect, such as in the treatment of ear, nose, and throat infections with antibiotics. Snuffs are solid medicine dose forms that are finely split and inhaled through the nostrils.

Examples include Braniff and Dentobac® Snuff.

Advantages:

1 The powder is sprayed by an insufflator into a stream of tiny particles that cover the area is applicable.

2. Create a local impact.

Disadvantages:

1 Difficulty in acquiring a precise dosage of the medication.

2. It becomes clogged when the powder is damp or is somewhat wet.

DENTRIFICES

Dentifrices (also known as tooth powders) are solutions that are typically applied to the teeth's surfaces along with a toothbrush. They come in the form of pastes and fine powders. They include a suitable detergent or soap, an abrasive material in the form of a fine powder, sodium as a sweetener, and a suitable flavour.

Examples include Close-up, Miswak, and Colgate Tooth Paste & Powder.

Advantages:

1. Dentifrices aid in maintaining healthy, clean teeth.

2. They exhale nicely.

3. They safeguard teeth against plaque, cavities, and gum illnesses.

4. Maintaining white teeth

Disadvantages:

1.Health problems are caused by the fluoride in toothpaste.

2.Flavored dentifrices are ineffective at preventing plaque.

3. They shield teeth from plaque, caries, and gum conditions.

4. Maintain teeth's whiteness

CACHETS

Rice paper disc- or cylinder-shaped objects called cachets have a lower and upper half, with the latter having a narrower flange. Between the two halves, the medication for unpleasant t is sealed. Cachets come in two varieties.

(1) Powdered medication is contained in the lower part of wet seal cachets. The bottom half of the cachet is then pressed over the wet flange of the empty upper half of the cachet. It takes 15 minutes to dry the cachet.

(ii) Dry seal cachets: The lower half is filled with drug powder, while the top half is sealed pressed like a capsule over it.

Examples include Isoniaze, Sodium Amino Salicylate, and Sodium Amino Salicylate Cachets.

Advantages

1. They are used to give drugs with bad tastes.

2. They are applied when a significant dose of the medication is administered.

Disadvantages:

1. Before administering, pre-use preparation is necessary. A cachet must be briefly submerged in water.

2. Complicated administration because it must be placed on the tongue and then swallowed water is used.

BEADS

The multi-particulate dose forms, called beads, can be contained inside an outer capsule shell and taken orally. A tablet dosage form can be created by compressing beads along with additional excipients.

Among them are Adderall XR® Beads. Mesoporous Methylphenidate.

PELLETS

It is possible to put these multi-particulate dose forms in an outer capsule shell for administration. To create a tabi dosage form, pellets can be compressed with additional excipients.

Examples include pellets of calcium chloride and plant extract.

Advantages:

1. Easy to dose and have superior flow behaviour are round pellets.

2. They are exceptionally stable, have a compact structure, good dispensability, high bulk density, and a dense surface.

3. They have a homogeneous surface, thin grain size, very low hygroscopicity, and are dense widespread and with little abrasion High active ingredient content are possible.

5. They are suitable for controlled-release applications and have the best starting form for additional coating.

6. Without a procedure or formulation, they can be separated into the necessary dosage strength.

7. Active component pellets in the form of suspension capsules or dissolving tablets have important therapeutic advantages over single unit dose forms.

8. By combining them, incompatible bioactive agents can be delivered. They can be utilised to offer various release profiles at the same or distinct places in a GIT.

10. Pellets provide a great degree of design and development flexibility for oral dosage forms such as solution, sachet, tablet, and capsule.

Disadvantages:

1. Dosing by volume rather than by number and, if necessary, dividing into single dose units.
2. Involves tableting, which damages film, or capsule filling, which might increase expenses pellets with coatings.
3. From formulation to formulation, particle size varies.
4. The potential for localised GI-tract mucosal injury.

VAGINAL RINGS

To distribute pharmaceuticals to the vagina in a controlled manner over a lengthy period of time, vaginal rings are doughnut-shaped polymeric drug delivery systems. As examples, Fem" Ring (estradiol-acetate) and Nuva" Ring (progesterone and estrogen).

INTRAUTERINE DEVICES

It is a coil or an IUD, a birth control method inserted into the uterus. The most used reversible birth control method in the world is the IUD. A doctor must insert the gadget into or remove it from the uterus. When pregnancy is not desired, it remains in place the entire time. A single IUD can be used for five to ten years, depending on the kind. IUDs fall into two general categories: inert, copper-based devices and hormonally-based devices that function via releasing progesterone.

SEMI-SOLID DOSAGE FORM

In simpler two-phase or multiphase systems, semisolid dosage forms are referred to as single-phase systems with the drug ingredient in solution in the semisolid material or medication.

Advantages:

1. It has an external use.
2 The likelihood of adverse effects is low.
3. Spent much of the time doing local action

Disadvantages:

1. This kind of dose form lacks dosing precision.
2. It is simple for the base utilised in the semi-solid dosage form to oxidise.
3. Issues may arise if we leave the house after taking semi-solid dosage form.

CREAMS

Designed for external use, creams are watery, greasy, viscous liquids or semisolid emulsions.

Examples include zinc cream, hydrocortisone cream, cetrimide cream, and cetomacrogol cream use BPC.

Advantages:

1. Because they are easier to apply and are less oily, creams are more acceptable.
2. They don't disrupt skin processes as much.
3. O/w creams are superior to w/o creams since they can be applied more readily and are simple to wash off.
4. Unflavored creams can be applied more evenly.
5. O/w creams are less prone to smear on clothing.
6. Cooling sensation is caused by water from o/w type of cream evaporating.
7. An o/w cream quickly absorbs liquid exudate that is discharged from a wound.
8. On prevent dehydration and irritation, w/o creams can be applied to non-weeping skin regain softness
9. Creams deliver hormones into the bloodstream precisely as intended.
10. May be utilised to prevent liver's first effects.

Disadvantages:

1. Creams should not be consumed internally.

2. Molds and bacteria can easily grow in the aqueous phase.
3. Preservatives are necessary to stop product deterioration.
4. Creams' oil components are vulnerable to rancidification.
5. A delayed start to activity.
6. Requires daily and intermittent application.
7. Extremely skinny persons might need to take their medication more frequently.

GELS

To apply externally to the skin or mucous membrane for lubrication or treatment, gels are transparent or non-greasy semisolid formulations.

Examples include Ichthammol jelly, contraceptive jelly (with spermicidal effect), and more. Gelatin is one of the gelie agents, however it can also be starch, tragacanth, sodium alginate, or a cellulose derivative.

Advantages:

1. First pass effects are avoided by using gels.
2. They have a lower risk of blood clotting than oral estrogens.
3. Gels contain more liquid than magma.
4. Because they are clear or translucent, non-greasy, semisolid gels, jellies are appealing.
5. They are utilised to lubricate rectal thermometers, surgical gloves, and catheters.

Disadvantages:

1. Gels start working more gradually.
2. They must be applied every day.
3. Dosing intervals must be increased.

OINTMENTS

Ointments are the oily, soft, semisolid, and soft formulations used externally on the skin or mucous membrane (rectum and nasal mucosa). Typically, they have a medication that has been dissolved, suspended, or emulsified in the base. Compound Benzoic Acid Ointment and Cetrimide Emulsifying Ointment are two examples.

Advantages:

1. Ointments are applied to the skin to provide emollient and protective properties.
2. Handling creams is simpler than handling large liquid dose forms.
3. They have a very low concentration of powdered particles.
4. When applied, they have a smooth feel and are soft.
5. They spread farther outside the treatment area because they are less viscous.
6. They are non-porous, therefore sweat cannot escape through them.
7. Compared to liquid dose forms, they are chemically more stable.

Disadvantages:

1. Compared to solid dosage forms, they are thicker.
2. It is challenging to apply the right amount of ointment to the injured area.
3. Compared to solid dose forms, they are less stable.

Ointments are divided into medicated and non-medicated categories.

PASTES

The firge Pastes are semisolid treatments intended to be applied topically to the skin. They typically contain significant amounts of finely powdered materials, such as calcium carbonate, zinc oxide, and starch.

Examples include pastes made of coal tar, zinc, and magnesium sulphate.

Advantages:

1. They give the regions where they are applied a protective coating.
2. They are effective as protective coatings due to their rigidity.
3. Pastes are less oily, penetrating, and macerating than liquids.
4. It creates an impermeable layer of film on the skin, and the substance it contains can absorb and neutralise some toxic compounds before they even get to the skin.

Disadvantages:

1.Are not as occlusive as creams (can be a benefit depending on indication).

2.Pastes frequently have pores that allow moisture to escape from the applied region because of their high solids content.

3. Pastes are typically placed in a thick coating where it is thought to be unattractive from a cosmetic standpoint.

4. The usage of pastes is frequently linked to clothing stains

5. Pastes' viscosity may make it difficult to evenly distribute the dosage form across the afflicted area.

Kaolin Poultice BPC, as an example.

LIQUID DOSAGE FORMS

It is meant to administer or consume a dose of a chemical compound used as a drug or medication in liquid form. Liquid dose forms may be routinely taken orally or injected using a variety of methods into the skin, muscles, or veins.

MIXTURES

A mixture is a dose form that combines two or more distinct chemicals physically rather than chemically. When two or more substances are physically combined, their identities are maintained, and the mixture takes the shape of suspensions or colloids.

Examples: Iromac XT Mixture (ferrous ascorbate folic acid)

SOLUTIONS

Solutions are liquid dosage forms that include one or more pharmacological substances dissolved in one or more solvents to create a transparent, homogeneous, single-phase system.

Advantages:

1. Solutions move more quickly.
2. They are simpler to digest.
3. They can change the dose with more freedom.

Disadvantages:

1. The shelf life of medicines in solutions are shorter.
2. The majority of solutions taste bad.
3. They can leak and are awkward to handle.
4. They need to be measured carefully.
5. Solutions need certain handling or storage needs.

INJECTABLES

For administration with a hypodermic (hollow-painted) needle, injectables are liquid formulations that can be made into liquids, powders, or lyophilized solutions.

Examples include Orfenac Injection (diclofenac) and Laennec® Injection (human placental extract)

(a) Irrigations: Wound irrigation solutions are used to hydrate the wound, remove debris and bacteria, facilitate visual inspection, prevent infection, enhance healing and cosmesis, and prevent infection. Saline solution is frequently used for wound irritation. sterile water that has been added with 1% povidone-iodine.

Examples include irrigation with 5% mannitol and 0.25% acetic acid.

b) Pharmaceutical injections: These fluids (solutions) are sterile and free of pyrogens packed in either single-dose or multidose containers, solid dosage forms (such as emulsions, suspensions, or solid dosage forms) containing one or more active Ingredients.

Examples include injections of carboplatin, midoryx (midazolam), and calcium gluconate.

Advantages:

1. Drugs that are poorly absorbed, inert, or ineffective when administered orally can be administered through injection.

2. Because there is no waiting period after receiving an intravenous injection, absorption.

3. To produce a delayed or sluggish onset of effect, use the i.m. and s.c. routes. 4. Issues with patient concordance can be avoided.

Disadvantages

1. Healthcare staff members require more training and evaluation.
2. Injections could be expensive.
3. They might hurt.
4. Injectables must be prepared using aseptic procedure.
5. They could need extra tools, including programmed infusion machines.

Infusions

Infusions (plasma-substituting preparations) are sterile, continuous-phase aqueous solutions. They are typically isotonic with regard to blood and free of pyrogens. They are given by infusion treatment, which entails giving medication through a catheter or needle. Typically, the term "infusion thera" refers to the administration of medication intravenously or subcutaneously. or emulsify more

Examples include Amphotercin B Infusion and Cloxatine Infusion (benzathine and cloxacillin).

Advantages:

1. Infusions are now offered as pre-filled, dose-specific items that are ready to use.
2. They come in hermetically sealed packaging for consistent sterility, better control, and cheaper overall costs.
3. They transport the medication directly into the bloodstream.

LOTIONS

Liquid preparations for friction-free exterior application are called lotions. To lessen evaporation, they are eit and dabbed on the skin or put to an appropriate dressing and covered with water proof material.

Examples include Salicylic Acid Lotion (dandruff), Salicylic Acid and Mercuric Chloride Lotion (ulcer), Zinc Sulfate and Salicylic Cas (impetigo), and Copper and Zinc Sulfate Lotion (impetigo) (follic Adv infection).

APPLICATIONS

Applications are viscous or liquid preparations meant to be applied to the skin. They are typically emulsions or suspensions. The majority of certified preparations are pesticides and have a finite number of applications. To distinguish them from preparations intended for shared use, they are distributed in coloured fluted bottles. For external use only is written on the container. cont

Case in point: lactocalamine

COLLODIONS

Collodions are liquid treatments designed to be applied topically to the skin. They are utilised when a prolonged contact between the skin and the medication is necessary and are practical for use on tiny cuts and abrasions. When applied to the skin, the vehicle evaporates, leaving a flexible, protective film that covers the area.

Examples include Mehran Collodion, Kryolam Collodion, and Collodium Collodion.

TINCTURES

These are alcohol-based formulations that contain the active ingredients of plant-based medications. They lack the strength of extracts. They can also be made by dissolving the equivalent liquid extract of a chemical compound (such as iodine) in alcohol or a hydroalcohol solvent. They are often made through maceration and percolation.

Examples are the tinctures of belladonna, aromatic cardamom, and iodine.

SPIRITS

Alcoholic or hydroalcoholic solutions of volatile chemicals are called spirits. The majority of spirits are used as flavourings, although some offer medical benefits.

Examples include compound orange spirit, lemon spirit, and chloroform spirit.

EMULSIONS

A liquid preparation known as an emulsion is essentially a mixture of water and oil that has been homogenised by the addition of an emulsifying agent. Only preparations meant for internal use are referred to as pharmaceutical emulsions. Emulsions for external usage are always given a different name that accurately describes their function, such as cream, lotion, or application. Emulsions can be divided into three categories: o/w, w/o, and w/o/w or o/w/o.

Examples include Castor Oil Emulsion, Liquid Paraffin Emulsion, Frelax® Oral Emulsion (magnesium hydroxide and liquid paraffin), and Fiatameal DS (aluminium hydroxide, magnesium hydroxide, and simethicone).

Advantages:

1. Unpleasant oils and unpalatable medications that are oil-soluble are delivered in palatable form using emulsions.
2. Emulsions can be easily flavoured in the aqueous phase.
3. It's simple to get rid of the greasy feeling.
4. A higher rate of medication absorption occurs.
5. Two incompatible ingredients can be used, one in each phase of the emulsion.

Disadvantages:

1. Before using, the emulsion preparation should be thoroughly shaken.
2. To administer emulsion, a measurement tool is required.
3. Measuring a dose requires a certain level of technical accuracy.
4. Emulsion stability may be impacted by storage conditions.
5. They are heavy, cumbersome, and prone to container breakages.
6. They can develop emulsio as a result of microbial infection cracking.

SUSPENSIONS

A pharmaceutical suspension is a coarse dispersion in which the external aqueous, organic, or oily liquid phase is uniformly distributed throughout the interior phase of insoluble solid particles with a particular range of size using a single or combination of agents lifting agent. Examples include Ceftef® Oral Suspension and Brufen Oral Suspension (ibuprofen) (cefixime)

Advantages:

1. Suspension can increase a drug's chemical stability.
2 The bioavailability of drugs in suspension is higher than that of other drugs.
3. Control over action's commencement and duration is possible.
4. Suspension can cover up the drug's harsh or bitter taste.

Disadvantages:

1. Sedimentation, compaction, and physical stability can all be problematic.
2. Susceptible to deterioration and potentially reactive to chemicals.

GASEOUS DOSAGE FORMS

Compressed medical gases can be supplied as a gas and come in gaseous and liquid (cryogenic) forms that are stored in high pressure cylinders. Fluids made expressly for the medical, pharmaceutical industry, and biotechnology sectors are known as pharmaceutical and medical gases. They are typically employed to create, sanitise, or insulate procedures or items that improve human health. Patients who receive gas therapy also breathe in pharmaceutical gases. Most frequently, a continuous-flow anaesthetic machine or a medical ventilator are used in medical facilities to inject gases into a patient's airway. Laryngeal masks, endotracheal tubes, and tracheostomy tubes are additional ways to get the gas into the patient's lungs.

Examples include medical air, oxygen, carbon dioxide, helium, nitrogen, and nitrous oxide.

AEROSOLS

An aerosol is defined as a disperse phase system in which very minute solid drug particles or liquid droplets are dispersed in a continuous propellant phase (gas).

Examples include Solarcaine Spray and fluoridated Oral B Foam (lidocaine)

Advantages:

1. The aerosol dose may be removed easily from the container without contamination.
2. Aerosols are simple and handy to use, and they can be administered alone.
3. When compared to other dose formulations, the beginning of effect is quicker.
4. The medication has excellent dispersion.
5. Drugs in aerosol form can avoid being broken down by enzymatic or pH action.

6. Drugs that are impacted by ambient oxygen or moisture may have their stability increased. intestinal or stomach.

7. Sterility of the products is preserved.

Disadvantages:

1. Aerosols are reasonably priced.
2. It is challenging to dispose of empty aerosol cans.
3. The propellant(s) can aggravate the skin damage due to their volatility.
4. In those who are sensitive to the propellant(s), repeated use may have a carcinogenic effect.
5. Aerosol packs must be kept away from heat and flames to prevent explosion.
6. It is challenging to create medications that are insoluble in propellant like aerosols.
7. Propellers may be toxic if therapy is sustained for an extended period of time reactions.

METHODIZED DOSE

An MDI, sometimes referred to as a metered-dosage inhaler, is a medical device that uses inhalation to deliver a precise dose of medication to the lungs in the form of a brief burst of aerosolized medication. For the treatment of respiratory conditions such asthma, chronic obstructive pulmonary disease (COPD), and others, it is the delivery modality that is used the most frequently. Bronchodilators and corticosteroids are most typically administered using metered dose inhalers to treat COPD and asthma.

Examples are QVAR (beclomethasone) and Ashtalin Inhalation (salbutamol sulphate BP).

INHALERS OF DRY POWDER

A dry powder inhaler is a small, portable device used to provide medications to the lungs while you breathe through it. There are no propellants or extra compounds used; only the medication is present.

For instance, Ventolin (salbutamol). Dry powder inhalers for Xopenex HFA (levalbuterol), Atrovent (ipratropium), and Pulmicort (budesonide). HFA.

IIMPORTANT QUESTIONS

Q1.Define drug. Give many medication sources.

Q2. Why did a dosage form need to be developed.

Q3. Describe dosage forms and classify them using examples.

QS4. Go over the benefits and drawbacks of various dose forms.

CHAPTER III

Prescription

With directions for palliation or the restoration of the patient's health, a prescription order between a doctor and patient is a crucial therapeutic transaction that highlights the doctor's therapeutic expertise and diagnostic aptitude. But if a prescription order doesn't communicate with the pharmacist clearly and doesn't adequately explain to the patient how to take the recommended drug, it could lose its therapeutic value. Thus, the objectives of this chapter are:

- Understanding the appropriate approach to handle a prescription.
- Improving prescription filling and refilling skills and learning how to write, read, and understand prescriptions.
- To underline the significance of writing prescriptions accurately. to raise awareness of the issues brought on by prescription writing mistakes and strategies to reduce them.
- To determine the prevalence or rate of prescription error and evaluate its causes,
- Devise creative interventions for the practitioners to stop medication mistakes.

Prescription

A prescription is an order written by a registered medical practitioner (RMP), doctor, dentist, or a veterinarian, etc to a pharmacist to compound and dispense the specified medication for the patient. The prescription acts as a conduit of shared interest between the patient, the doctor, and the pharmacy. The prescription serves as a vehicle for communicating a treatment modality to the patient in the form of written instructions. Each patient's prescription is a special document that specifies a certain drug or medications for a particular patient at a particular time.

The prescription is typically written on paper, but it can now be printed on a particular form. The form has vacant spaces where the required information can be filled in. The doctors are frequently given these blanks in the form of a pad comprising 100 blank forms.

The order accompanies the directions for the pharmacist as to what type of preparation is to be prepared, as well as directions for the patient regarding the dosage and frequency of the administration. The pharmacist must maintain and respect the confidentiality of the patient in context to their illness and nature of treatment.

Earlier, medicines were prescribed in Latin language, but now-a-days they are written in the language of the area in which they originate. Still the use of Latin abbreviations can be frequently observed in the dosage instructions. For the best possible communication between the prescriber, pharmacist, and nurse, all prescription orders must be accurate, clear, without cross-outs, and signed in large letters.

Functions of a Prescription

1. One may utilise a prescription as a legal document.
2. It might be a source of records.
3. It serves as a tool for communicating.
4. It is required when using a therapeutic approach.
5. It is a method of therapeutic treatment control.
6. It is a clinical trial tool.

Parts of a Prescription

A medically correct and complete prescription should include the following parts: -

1. Prescriber's details
2. Details of the patient
3. Superscription
4. Inscription

5. Subscription
6. Signatura/Transcription/Signa
7. Renewal
8. Signature
9. Other important instructions

1. **Prescriber's details**: - Details about the prescriber include the doctor's first and last names, the hospital, clinic, or polyclinic where they receive care, their address, the doctor's name, title, registration number, phone number, e-mail address, and the date. The ability to contact the doctor in an emergency to get clarification, necessary instructions, confirmation, etc., depends on having information on the doctor. A prescription number is necessary for insurance or refill purposes. The date is significant in terms of determining how long the prescription will last. The prescriber must include the date on the prescription at the same time as the writing. When a prescription is brought in for dispensing years after it was issued, the date on the prescription helps the pharmacist identify these instances. Unlike orders for children, which can be renewed seven days after the original date of issuance, prescriptions for narcotics and prohibited drugs cannot be filled after more than ten days from the date of issuance due to particular rules and restrictions. As a result, the date must be on any prescriptions for narcotics or other habit-forming medications.
2. **Details of the patient**: - The patient's name, address, age, and sex are all listed in this section of the prescription. Instead of only the surname or the family name, the patient's full name must be written. This information is required to be written on the prescription since it aids in its identification. The pharmacist should ask the patient about these specifics and note the information at the top of the prescription if it is not already written there. Only the patient whose name appears on the prescription is allowed to take the prescribed drug. Even if the patients share identical symptoms, it is still inappropriate to administer medications to another patient. This eliminates the chance of giving the final item to someone other than the intended recipient. The patient's age and gender, particularly in the case of children, aid the pharmacist in determining the prescription and dosage. As a result, there will be less chance that the wrong family member or that a hospital ward with a similar name will receive it. Age and weight are crucial factors in the calculation of the dose, dose frequency, and delivery route. The patient's address is kept on file in case it's needed later for reference, to get in touch with the patient, or to personally deliver the medication.
3. **Superscription**: - The detailed instructions for the pharmacist on how to mix the medication are included in a superscription. The Rx symbol, which is always written at the start of the prescription, stands in for the superscription. In the days of mythology and superstition, the symbol was interpreted as a supplication to Jupiter, the God of healing, for the patient's speedy recovery. However, nowadays, this symbol is recognised as an acronym for the Latin word recipe, which means "take thou" or "you take." The majority of directions are typically expressed using abbreviations or contracted Latin. Additionally, there are preparation instructions like "create a mixture," "mix and form 10 pills," or "dispense 10 capsules."
4. **Inscription**: - It is the main part of the prescription. It contains the names of the medication, or the quantities of the ingredients prescribed. In a complex prescription, the inscription is presented in three parts,

a) the active constituent, that is intended to produce the therapeutic action,

b) the adjuvant, which either enhances the efficacy of the active medicament or serves the purpose of making it more palatable,

c) the vehicle, it is incorporated in the formulation for dissolving the solids or to increase the quantity of the finished product for ease in administration.

Additionally, the prescriber takes enough care of the following three components.

1. Use of a generic name or a trademark name (INN - international non-proprietary name). The medical drugs must be in the Genitive case and have a capital letter at the start.

2. The dosage form is either listed before or after the name of the medicine.

3. Following the name of the medication comes a dose notation. The medication's strength is specified in metric units.

Example: Tab. Ibuprofen.... 600 mg.

Now-a-days the medications are already formulated into dosage forms by the industrial manufacturers, eliminating the compounding of prescription by the pharmacists.

5. **Subscription**: - It contains directions for the pharmacist by the prescriber regarding the type of dosage form and the number of doses to be dispensed. As only few prescriptions are compounded by the pharmacists now-a-days, hence such directions are rarely used.
6. **Signatura**: - It is abbreviated as 'Sig' on the prescription and contains instructions for the patient in context to the administration of the medicament, quantity, number, or dosage units to be taken, time and manner of administration or application. The pharmacist should transfer these directions on the label of the container and ensure that the patient complies to it carefully. Despite the fact that the Signatura should always be written in English, some doctors nevertheless use Latin abbreviations. For example,
7. '1 Cap t.i.d. pc' is translated into English as "take one capsule three times each day, following meals".
8. '1 Tab t.i.d.' means "one tablet three times a day".

7. **Renewal**: - The doctor specifies in the renewal instructions how often a prescription is to be repeated. Along with any additional instructions or cautions, it may also include the prescriber's signature, which is often that of a doctor.
8. **Signature**: - The prescriber's name should be handwritten and signed with ink, for authenticating the prescription. It also eliminates the danger of dispensing any medicament on spurious order. The prescriber's address and registration number must be visible on any prescriptions for narcotics or other habit-forming medications. This specifies the unique licence that a doctor needs in order to write prescriptions for narcotics and other habit-forming medications.

9. **Other important instructions**: -

(a) Refills: The prescription needs to specify the number of refills allowed or whether they're prohibited.

(b) Qty: The "quantity" or amount of the package.

(c) Mfg... "Manufacturer" or the person who creates the drug.

(d) Expiration date: After this time, the drug should not be used. Don't keep unused medicines. If the same patient becomes ill once more, the prescriber should be contacted. (e) Complete the course of treatment: Patients who are receiving antibiotics should finish taking the entire prescription, even if they feel better. This prevents infection recurrence and the emergence of resistance.

(f) Take with/without food: Indicates whether to take the drug on an empty stomach or after a meal. While certain medications operate better when the stomach is empty, others do better when it is full.

(g) Four times a day refers to taking the drug four times in a 24-hour period at evenly spaced intervals. Compared to Take every four hours, it is different. If there is any doubt regarding when to provide the pills, one should speak with a doctor or pharmacist. Although certain prescriptions require exact timing, the majority don't.

(h) Take as needed as long as symptoms last: This means that you can take the drug whenever you have symptoms without first talking to your doctor.

(i) Additional informational warning labels in vivid colours may also be present on the box. Here are several examples:

1. Directions for secure storage, such as "keep refrigerated."
2. Instructions like "shake well before use."
3. Adverse effects that could occur, including "may cause drowsiness."

A layman may find it challenging to interpret and comprehend prescriptions. Even a beginning pharmacist needs to put in some work and undergo training. He only reads the prescription after gaining a great deal of experience. The busy doctor always writes quickly and uses a lot of abbreviations, which a pharmacist must understand alone. Doctors frequently have a reputation for having poor handwriting that is difficult to read. It is customary for prescriptions to be written quickly at times and in Latin. Latin is no longer taught in most medical and pharmacy curriculum these days. Doctors still commonly utilise Latin terminology and abbreviations because they have very deep roots. In reality, in the past, a patient's prescription was a mystery and kept a secret between the doctor and the pharmacy. There is no longer a need for secrecy due to rising drug knowledge and easy access to drug-related information. As a result, the patient has a right to know what medication has been given, and the Consumer Protection Act protects his interests.

Prescription Types

There are two types of prescriptions: Compounded and Non-compounded.

1. **Compounded prescription:** Extemporaneous prescriptions are another name for compounded prescriptions. It is a request that one or more medications be combined with one or more pharmaceutical excipients. The pharmacist makes the medication in accordance with the medications, doses, and dosage forms chosen by the doctor. Each drug's name is listed on a separate line beneath the one that comes before it.
2. **Non-compounded prescription:** A non-compounded prescription does not need to have two or more ingredients mixed together to create the final product. When a pharmaceutical business supplies a medicine or combination of drugs under its legal or proprietary name, it is known as a pre-compounded order. If the order comprises more than one substance, the precise ingredients do not need to be mentioned.

Units of measurement used in prescriptions

Drug potency should be expressed in metric units. Drug dosages are expressed in grams, milligrams, and micrograms. The fundamental unit of weight in the metric system is the gram (g). Milligrams are one thousandth of a gram (mg). One microgram (g) or one mcg is one thousandth of a milligram. One kilogram is equal to 1000 grams. In the metric system, the litre serves as the fundamental unit of volume. The millilitre (ml), which is one thousandth of a litre, is a unit that is frequently used. As a unit equivalent to millilitres, the cubic centimetre, or cc, is used. The amount of a solute in solvent to make 100 ml is typically used to express the strength of a solution.

For example, A 100 ml (g/100 ml) of potassium chloride solution (20% KCl) contains 20 grams of KCl. One millilitre of distilled water at 4 degrees Celsius in vacuum equals one gram.

Handling of Prescription

As soon as a patient enters the pharmacy, they should feel welcomed and at ease through courteous gestures and a welcoming environment. Open lines of communication should enable the patient to express his or her demands by presenting a prescription or by requesting more advice or goods.

1. When the pharmacist receives the prescription, they should confirm the patient's identity and whether they are the ones handing over the prescription or whether someone else is.

2. The patient may be kindly asked to wait while the pharmacist examines the prescription for therapeutic factors, including pharmaceutical and pharmacological dosages suited for the patient, social, legal, and economic considerations, as well as the prescription's legality and completeness.

3. The doctor's name, address, and registration number should all be included on the prescription, along with the patient's name, address, age, sex, height, and weight, as well as the name(s), potency, dosage, and total number of medications to be given. The prescription should also include instructions for the patient, refill information, if applicable, and the doctor's usual signature.

Any ambiance, perplexity, flaw, or anomaly should be brought to the prescribing doctors' attention.

The prescription should be checked for the following:

1. Dosage: Determine whether the prescribed dosage falls within the acceptable minimum and maximum range.

2. Double medicine: When more than one doctor is treating the same patient concurrently, double medication (either the same drug or a different drug with the same pharmaco-therapeutic effect) is prescribed by the same doctor or two different doctors.
3. Interaction: Any interactions between the patient's current prescription drugs, over the counter (OTC) drugs, and drugs from any previous prescriptions (records of which may be found in the patient's medication records). The prescribing clinician should be informed of any drug interactions that could make the therapy ineffective or have unfavourable consequences on the patients.
4. Contraindication: A patient's age, sex, disease(s), condition(s), or other traits that may make some of their prescribed medications contraindicated.
5. History: History of the patient misusing or abusing their medications.

Any of the aforementioned issues, together with any handwriting readability issues, should be brought to the prescribing Doctors' attention. Changes made over the phone in consultation with the Dr. (name) at (time) on (date) should be noted on the prescription with the words "Changes made over the telephone in consultation with the Dr. (name)". If in doubt, get the prescription from the prescribing doctor and have it suitably adjusted. This activity demands a professional, trust-based relationship with the prescribing doctor..

Errors in Prescription

A drug or prodrug is typically referred to as a medication (a medicinal product) since it contains an active pharmaceutical ingredient. Contaminants may also be present in medication. a biologically active component plus excipients, or just excipients. One which is meant to be consumed by or given to a human or animal for any of the mentioned purposes is considered as an active medicinal product:

1. As a substitute (placebo);
2. Prevent an illness;
3. Make a diagnosis;
4. Check for any potential negative effects;
5. Alter an anomaly or physiological, biochemical, or anatomical function:
6. Replace a lacking component;
7. Reduce a symptom;
8. Cure an illness;
9. Elicit anaesthesia.

The act of administering a drug to a patient is known as medication (the procedure), and it might be done for any of these reasons.

An error

An error is defined as "anything done incorrectly due to ignorance or accident; a mistake." For instance, "a failure to finish planned action as intended, or the implementation of an improper plan of action to attain a particular purpose," in calculation, judgement, speaking, writing, action, etc.

A medication error

Medication error can be described as "a failure in the therapeutic process that causes, or has the potential to cause, harm to the patient." Drug errors can occur during the prescription process, the dispensing process, the administration of the medication, or the patient compliance process.

Medication Error Types

Type	Definition
Prescribing error	Incorrect medication selection (based on indications, contraindications, known allergies, existing drug therapy, and other considerations), dosage, dosage form, route, concentration, administration, or usage instructions of a prescription product ordered or authorised by a physician (or other valid prescriber); prescriptions or medication orders that are not legible and cause errors to be delivered to the patient
Omission error	The inability or failure to give a patient an contract/ordered dose prior to their next, if any, scheduled dose
Wrong time error	Administration of a medicine outside of the window of time designated for its administration
Unauthorised drug error	Administration of medication to the patient without authorization from a valid prescriber for the patient
Improper dose error	Delivery of duplicate doses, i.e., one or more dosage units over and above the prescribed number, or administration of a dose to the patient that is either greater than or less than the quantity the physician requested
Wrong dosage-form error	Administration of a medication in a dosage form other than that specified by the doctor
Wrong drug preparation error	Drug preparation that was fabricated or altered improperly before use
Wrong administration technique error	Incorrect approach or process used for administering a medication
Deteriorated drug error	Administering a medicine which has surpassed the expiry date or whose dosage form authenticity is compromised in either its physical or chemical composition
Monitoring error	Inability to properly analyse a given procedure to ensure suitability and issue identification, or disregard for suitable medical or experimental (laboratory) data for effective evaluation of the patient's response to the recommended treatment
Compliance error	Improper patient behaviour when it comes to taking ordered medications as directed
Other medication error	Any pharmaceutical error not specifically mentioned in the list above

Type
Definition
Prescribing error

Incorrect medication selection (based on indications, contraindications, known allergies, existing drug therapy, and other considerations), dosage, dosage form, route, concentration, administration, or usage instructions of a prescription product ordered or authorised by a physician (or other valid prescriber); prescriptions or medication orders that are not legible and cause errors to be delivered to the patient

Omission error

The inability or failure to give a patient an contract/ordered dose prior to their next, if any, scheduled dose

Wrong time error

Administration of a medicine outside of the window of time designated for its administration

Unauthorised drug error

Administration of medication to the patient without authorization from a valid prescriber for the patient

Improper dose error

Delivery of duplicate doses, i.e., one or more dosage units over and above the prescribed number, or administration of a dose to the patient that is either greater than or less than the quantity the physician requested

Wrong dosage-form error

Administration of a medication in a dosage form other than that specified by the doctor

Wrong drug preparation error

Drug preparation that was fabricated or altered improperly before use

Wrong administration technique error

Incorrect approach or process used for administering a medication

Deteriorated drug error

Administering a medicine which has surpassed the expiry date or whose dosage form authenticity is compromised in either its physical or chemical composition

Monitoring error

Inability to properly analyse a given procedure to ensure suitability and issue identification, or disregard for suitable medical or experimental (laboratory) data for effective evaluation of the patient's response to the recommended treatment

Compliance error

Improper patient behaviour when it comes to taking ordered medications as directed

Other medication error

Any pharmaceutical error not specifically mentioned in the list above

Prevention of Medication error

The classification of medication errors—which might be contextual, modal, or psychological—can help us understand how they occur and how to prevent them. Contextual classification takes into account the precise moment, location, substances, and participants. Modal classification investigates how errors happen (for example, by omission, repetition or substitution). It is preferable to categorise things psychologically since it explains happenings as opposed to just describing them. The fact that it focuses more on human error than rational error is a drawback. There are primarily four categories of medication error.

1. **Knowledge-based errors**: Issues with top staff communication and acquiring the right medication. Dosing details played a role in knowledge-based prescription errors. Example. providing penicillin without first determining whether the patient is allergic These mistakes ought to be preventable by being knowledgeable about the medication being recommended and the patient to whom it is being administered. Such errors can be prevented with the aid of computerised prescribing/ordering systems, bar-coded drug systems, and cross-checking by pharmacists and nurses. A good education is crucial.
2. **Rule-based errors**: Mistakes based on rules (employing an erroneous rule or a good rule incorrectly). For instance, administering diclofenac into the lateral thigh as opposed to the buttock. These kinds of errors can be prevented with the use of appropriate guidelines, education, and computerised prescribing/ordering systems.

3. **Action-based rules (Slips):** For instance, choosing quinine from the shelf rather than quinidine. The majority of mistakes, it has been shown, are the result of carelessness during normal prescription, administering drugs or distributing. It could be reduced by establishing circumstances in which they are less likely to occur (e.g., by staying focused and double-checking, by properly labelling medications, and by utilising identifiers, like bar-codes, which has been proposed as a way to avoid label misreading). The technical error is a subset of action-based faults, such as incorporating the incorrect quantity of potassium chloride into an infusion bottle. Use of checklists, fail-safe systems and computerised reminders can be helpful in reducing these types of errors.
4. **Memory-based errors (Lapses):** Memory-based errors are challenging to prevent, but they can be stopped through cross-checking and computerised prescribing systems. As an illustration, imagine administering penicillin despite knowing the patient has an allergy.

Potential error

A potential error is a mistake made when a drug is prescribed, dispensed, or planned to be administered that is discovered and fixed through action before the medication is actually administered. To find possibilities to address issues in the pharmaceutical use system even before they arise, potential mistakes are examined and categorised as distinct events from occurrence mistakes. Potential error detection is a typical step in the hospital's quality improvement approach. Documenting instances in which someone successfully avoided a medication error helps to highlight flaws in the system and emphasises the value of various checks in the medication use system.

Latent factors

'Active failures' refer to mistakes (errors based on knowledge and rule), slips (action or behaviour based errors), and lapses (errors based on memory). Prescribers are vulnerable to error due to a number of "latent variables." For instance, working overtime with minimal resources, poor support, and a precarious employment all raised the chance of prescription errors among nurses. Depression and tiredness are significant factors for doctors. Errors are more likely to happen when work is done after hours by harried, disoriented employees, frequently in the presence of new patients. Due to knowledge gaps and possibly also because they are unfamiliar with the local prescription charts and other systems, there is a higher chance of mistakes when doctors first enter a hospital. A national prescription form would be helpful. Better education and working conditions, particularly better induction procedures, should lower the probability of errors caused by these factors.

Detecting and reporting errors

One of the main challenges in identifying errors is the pharmacist who makes them dread disciplinary actions and do not want to report them, which could be avoided by opting for a non-punitive, blame-free environment at workplace. The informing of errors, especially close calls, should be encouraged. Error reports can be used to pinpoint locations where errors are most likely to occur, and the steps in the treatment process should be made simpler and more uniform. Some systems for voluntarily reporting medical errors, nevertheless, are only marginally beneficial since reports frequently lack specifics and are incomplete or underreported. Utilizing a variety of techniques may improve the detection of medication mistakes. A reporting method for these errors should be easily accessible, along with detailed instructions on how to submit a drug error, which should be followed by feedback.

Prescribing faults and prescription errors

Irrational prescription and improper prescribing are two categories of prescribing errors. prescription writing errors, ineffective prescribing, both under- and over-prescribing, etc. It is clear that the word "mistake" does not adequately characterise any of these. Errors other than mistakes committed when writing a prescription include failure in prescribing an anticoagulant for a patient to whom it is appropriate (under prescribing) or prescribing when it is not necessary or indicated (overprescribing). It is therefore suggested to use the words "prescription errors" and "prescriptive defects." Both of these forms are ambiguously included under the umbrella phrase "prescribing mistakes."

1. **Prescribing faults**

According to the Oxford English Dictionary, the terms "rational" and "appropriate" refer to something that is "specially fitted or fitting, proper." Although logical prescription should always be appropriate, this is not always the case. If a logical approach is founded on incomplete or inaccurate data, it may lead to inappropriate prescribing. A prescription for paracetamol might be reasonable yet improper, for instance, if the patient is unaware that another doctor has already tried paracetamol for a headache without result.

2. **Ineffective prescribing**

It is different from under prescribing to prescribe a medication that is ineffective for the patient or for the indication as a whole. Six percent of 1621 medicines were deemed unsuccessful in a research including 212 individuals. 112 (57%) of the 196 US out-patients 65 years and older who were taking five or more drugs did so because the medication was ineffective, inappropriate, or redundant. And in a Scottish study, 5% of practises prescribed 50% of the homoeopathic treatments, which were prescribed in 49% of general practises. The implementation of guidelines should reduce ineffective prescribing, however there is conflicting research that suggests they may not be as effective without additional support from education or financial incentives.

3. **Under prescribing**

Under prescribing is the use of an inappropriately low dose of an appropriate drug or the neglect to prescribe an acceptable and suggested medication. Although the full incidence of under prescribing is unknown, there is evidence of severe under prescribing of some highly effective medicines, like statins for hyperlipidaemia and angiotensin converting enzyme inhibitors for patients with heart failure. Fear of interaction-related side effects, a failure to acknowledge the necessity of therapy, and uncertainty or ignorance regarding the likelihood of success are some of the causes of under prescribing. Cost might be a factor. Age may have a role in the tendency for older people to delay treatment, which might have unintended consequences such as the so-called risk-treatment mismatch, when those who are most at risk receive less aggressive care. Other issues, such as co-morbidities distracting patients, underestimating the true benefit versus harm of balancing, and reluctance to start or worsen multiple pharmacological therapy are all possible causes of this kind mismatch.

4. **Overprescribing**

Overprescribing is when a medicine is prescribed in an excessive dosage (too much, too often or for too long). Sometimes, medical intervention is completely unnecessary. For instance, just half of hospital patients who received a proton pump inhibitor medication were considered to be in need of it. Over 10% of people over 65 years age have polypharmacy, which is defined as the use of five or more medicines.. While not all polypharmacy is bad, some of it unquestionably causes ADRS and drug-drug interactions. Antibiotic overuse is a widely known and debated topic.

5. **Prescription errors**

Prescription errors are generally a result of all the factors that cause pharmaceutical errors. Among them are ignorance, the use of an inaccurate medicine name, dose form, or abbreviation, as well as improper dosage calculations. A study found that 30% of medication errors in children's prescriptions, 25% of medication errors in dispensing, and 40% of medication errors in administration. The erroneous dose was recorded as the most frequent prescription error in one study. Improperly written patient's name and writing the erroneous dosage combination was responsible for 50% of all prescription chart errors in hospitals.

Achieving balanced prescribing

In the lack of data showing that using this schedule enhances prescription, it makes sense to utilise it. Each of the items listed below refers to an essential step in the prescribing process. Before issuing a prescription, the following nine inquiries should be made:

1. **Indication**: Does the medication have an indication?
2. **Effectiveness:** Does the prescribed drug work to treat the illness?
3. **Diseases:** Are there significant co-morbidities which could alter or impact how well a medicine works?
4. **Other similar drugs**: Are there any further medications the patient is taking that have similar effects?
5. **Interactions:** Does any clinically significant drug interactions between the patient's other medications exists?
6. **Dosage**: What is the ideal dosing schedule in terms of dose, frequency, route, and formulation?
7. **Orders**: Are the recommended dosage instructions for the medication practical?
8. **Period**: How long should a patient receive therapy?
9. **Economics**: Is the medication economical?

The five prescription writing standards below can help you write better prescriptions and decrease pharmaceutical errors.

1. Take education classes as often as you can (a repeat prescription-learning should be lifelong).
2. Graduates and undergraduates are obliged to take certain study modules as needed.
3. Proper evaluation; to be taken once or twice in the final undergraduate test; taken occasionally in postgraduate appraisal; it can be connected to a prescription drug licence.
4. A consistent, national hospital prescription form that will serve as a teaching aid.
5. Computerized prescribing systems and recommendations: to be followed where appropriate (the roles and proper implementation).

Some commonly used Latin Terms and Abbreviations in Prescriptions

Latin term or Phrase	Abbreviation	English meaning
Ad libitum	ad. lib.	As desired, at pleasure
Admove	admov.	Apply
Agita	agit.	Stir, shake
Alternis horis	alt. hrs.	Alternate hours
Ante cibos	a.c.	Before meals
Applicandus	applicand	To be applied
Aqua	aq.	Water
Bis in die	b.i.d.	Twice a day
Cibos	cibos.	Meals, food
Cum	c	With
Diebus alternis	dieb. alt.	Every other day
Dolore urgente	dol. urg.	When the pain is severe
E	-	With

E. lacte	e. lact.	With milk
Ex. aqua	ex. aq.	With water
Inter cibos	i.c.	During meals
Mistura	mist.	A Mixture
Omni hora	omn. hor. o.h.	Every hour
Parti affecti applicandus	p.a.a.	Apply at the afflicted or affected area
Phiala prius agitata	p.p.a.	Attach a 'shake the bottle first' label
Post cibos	p.c.	After meals
Quantum sufficiat	q.s.	As much as sufficient
Quarter in die	q.i.d.	Four times a day
Recipe	Rx	Take
Si opus sit	s.o.s.	When necessary
Statim	stat.	Immediately
Ter in die	t.i.d.	Three times a day

NAME OF HOSPITAL/CLINIC

Name of the Doctor/RMP

Qualifications (MBBS, MD, etc)

Registration No. ....

Address. ....

Contact No. .... Email ID. ....

Date: ../../..

Name of the Patient:	Age:	Sex:	Height:	Weight: .....
Address:	Contact No.		Email ID:	

℞

1. Name of medicine 1 (Quantity, Strength, Dosage instructions, Administration instructions)
2. Name of medicine 2 (Quantity, Strength, Dosage instructions, Administration instructions)

Other specific instructions (Drug interactions, precautions, etc)

Doctor's Signature Stamp

Dispensed by:

Date: ../../.. Name of Pharmacist: ....

Name of Pharmacy: .... Address: ....

CHAPTER IV

POSOLOGY

Posology is a field of medicine that deals with the dosage of medication that should be given to a patient in order to achieve the desired pharmacological effect. Bringing medication plasma concentration within the therapeutic window is the goal of drug therapy. The following are some of the chapter's goals:

- To research medicine dosages, particularly when it comes to choosing the right ones.
- To collect pertinent data to inform the posology suggestion while taking into consideration patient and product specifics.
- To recognise and comprehend the variables influencing medicine dosages. to be aware of the various dose calculating techniques for paediatric patients.

Posology

The term 'Posology' is a conjugation of two Greek words, 'Posos' which means 'how much' and 'Logos' which means science. Hence, it can be characterised as the area of medical research that deals with the amount or doses of medications that can be given to an individual to get a desired meaningful pharmacological reaction. In simple terms, it is the science of dose or dosage.

Dose: - The dose of a drug can be defined as the amount administered or consumed by the patient which is 'enough, but not too much', in order to produce the optimum therapeutic action. The idea is to induce maximum therapeutic benefit with the minimum possible dose. The dose is generally represented as a range rather than a fixed standard. The minimum dose is necessary to fabricate the required pharmacological action whereas the maximum dose is the largest amount that can be administered without producing any toxic effect in the patient.

Several cardinal factors such as age, severity of disease, condition of the patient, tolerance, idiosyncrasy, route of administration, bioavailability, and rate of elimination influence the dose of drug. Thus, the dose cannot be fixed rigidly or standardised for a particular drug.

Factors affecting Dose of a drug: -

There are various factors that affect the dose and action of a drug in an individual. They are mentioned as follows:

-

1. **Age**: - The age of an individual plays a significant role in determining the dose specially in children and elderly patients. The children below 12 years of age are given only a fraction of adult dose (16-80 years).

a. **New-borns:** - New-borns are particularly susceptible to some medicaments due to their underdeveloped or immature renal and hepatic system. The dosage is low because GIT secretions, liver microsomal enzymes (glucuronyl transferase) are not adequate, less protein binding, glomerular filtration rate and tubular secretions. Penicillin, streptomycin, and amino glycosides are not administered in children. Drug accumulation in the body can lead to toxicity and adverse effects.

b. **Children:** - Up to the age of 8, the child's dose is derived from the adult dose. The tissues of an infant and child require fewer doses since they are highly sensitive to large number of drugs. The drug metabolizing enzyme system is inefficient in the children under 12 years age (Glucuronidation takes 3 months to develop). The blood brain barriers (BBB) is not fully developed in children thus they are more sensitive to CNS stimulants. Tetracyclines can discolour teeth permanently, corticosteroids can stunt growth and development, and antihistamines can make kids hyperactive. Children can tolerate a relatively larger dosage of belladonna or digitalis on account of their body weight in comparison to adults.

c. Adult: - The average adult dose is designed for an individual of age 18-60 years with a minimum weight of 70 kg. The dose can be modified for obese or underweight patients.
d. Geriatric: - The geriatric patients belong to age group more than 60 years. Age-related physiological changes, like decreased weight of the body, decreased body-fat, decreased motility of the intestine and mesenteric blood flow, decreased live and kidney functions, and changed mental processes, necessitate specific attention for these individuals. Less medication is needed in elderly people as a result of renal and hepatic impairment brought on by ageing. Because they are more likely to have pharmacological side effects, seniors frequently need lower doses than adults.

5. **Sex**: - There is a possibility that females do not react to medications in the same manner as men. They require a lesser dose than men either due to their body weight or for being more responsive to certain drugs. Autonomic drug susceptibility is higher in females (oestrogen inhibits choline esterase). Prolactin levels may rise as a result of ulcer medication. Salicylates and potent purgatives should be avoided during menstruation since they may cause more bleeding. During lactation, some purgatives, penicillin, chloramphenicol, and oral anticoagulants may be excreted through milk and may have an impact on the baby. While morphine often causes CNS depression, some people, particularly women, may experience excitement when using it.
6. **Pregnancy**: - During pregnancy, heart rate, Glomerular Filtration Rate (GFR), renal medication elimination, volume of distribution, and metabolic rate of pharmaceuticals are considered. Lipophilic medications slowly exit the body after crossing the placental barrier. Uterine stimulants, potent purgatives, and medications that could have teratogenic effects should all be avoided during pregnancy. This is especially true during the first trimester, when no medication should be used unless it is absolutely essential. Morphine shouldn't be used during labour since it passes the placental barrier and impairs the breathing of new-born.
7. **Body weight**: - The general recommended adult doses are based on the standard body weight '70 kg'. But such a dose would be too less for an obese or muscular person and too large for a thin person. The dose calculated according to body weight is represented as mg/kg. Children dose calculated according to the body weight is considered more dependable.
8. **Route of administration**: - The therapeutic effectiveness of a drug highly depends on its route of delivery and the dosage form. Drugs given through the intravenous route show maximum bioavailability, hence lesser dose is sufficient, but also possess a higher risk of toxicity. Whereas drugs given through the oral route, require a higher dose to be administered because of multiple obstacles to their absorption such as the first pass metabolism. Drug absorption rates typically decline with mode of administration in the following order: intravenously > intramuscularly > subcutaneously > orally. Example: The dosage of ergotamine for the oral route is 2 to 5 mg, the intramuscular route is 1 mg (about 1/2 of the oral dose), and the intravenous route is 0.25 mg (roughly 1/8 of the oral dose and % of the intravenous dose).
9. **Time of administration**: - The key element determining how frequently a medicine should be administered is the biological half-life of the drug (the amount of time needed for the blood level to fall to 50% of the initial peak level). Example: Sulphadiazine has a biological half-life of 4 hours, necessitating the administration of 1 g of the medication every 4 hours following the initial dose of 2 g. Contrarily, the biological half-life of a medicine, such as the sedative reserpine, has no bearing on how frequently it is administered.
10. **Food**: - A drug which is effective when taken before meal gets readily absorbed on an empty stomach rather than a drug advised after meal. Drugs which are irritant in nature should be administered after meal to dilute its concentration. For e.g., iron, arsenic, cod liver oil, etc should be taken on a full stomach to reduce the gastric irritation.
11. **Environmental factors:** - Darkness is a psychological sedative, hence the amount of barbiturate needed to induce sleep during the day is higher than that at night. Stimulating drugs are more effective during the day whereas hypnotic drugs are more effective during night-time. Also, the tolerance for alcohol is more in colder environment as compared to summer.

12. **Emotional factors:** - The faith put by the patient in the doctor also plays a key role in medication. Nervous patients require lesser dose as compared to the normal ones. Bronchial asthma and angina pectoris have been treated successfully in some patients by placebo effect. Females are generally emotional and more responsive to drugs, thus require a lesser dosage than male to produce the same desired effect.
13. **Severity of disease:** - One aspirin tablet is frequently enough to ease a dull headache, but two to three of the same tablet may be required to treat a severe headache. However, this is not always the case. For instance, in the event of anaemia due to a lack of iron. The amount of iron that can be absorbed from the intestine daily and incorporated into haemoglobin is limited, hence the dose of iron salt that is given orally stays the same regardless of severity.
14. **Pathological state:** - If the organs that biotransformation or excretion occurs through are unhealthy, a lower dose is advised. For instance, phenobarbitone, which is primarily eliminated by the kidneys, is given in lesser doses in cases of renal insufficiency, and morphine is given in reduced doses to patients with liver problems (morphine is mainly inactivated in liver). Although aspirin lowers body temperatures in patients who are feverish, it has no effect on normal body temperature. Black water fever is more frequently precipitated by quinine when falciparum malaria is present than not. Similarly, patient suffering from liver cirrhosis might experience long lasting effect from certain drugs such as chlorpromazine and barbiturates.
15. **Accumulation:** - Repetitive administration of a drug for a long time can cause its unexpected accumulation leading to toxic effects. Cumulative effects are generally produced by slow elimination, unexpected rapid absorption, or improper degradation of drugs. Thus, drugs such as digitalis, emetine, heavy metals should be administered carefully.
16. **Plasma protein binding:** - Malnutrition reduces the amount of proteins and amino acids, which reduces the number of drug binding sites.

Simultaneous administration drugs: -

a. **Synergism:** -When two or more drugs are used together in a combined form and their effects are enhanced together, the phenomenon is called as synergism. E.g., the combination therapy of procaine with adrenaline, increases the effect of procaine. Synergism is helpful when the desired pharmacological effect of a drug is required in a single dose, and if the drug produces side effects at a relatively higher dose. Synergism is of two types:

i. **Addition:** An additive effect occurs when the combined effects of two or more medications are equal to the sum of each of those effects. E.g., ephedrine and aminophylline in the treatment of asthma.
ii. **Potentiation:** When the combined effect of two or more drugs is more than the sum of their individual effects, it is known as potentiation. E.g., the combination of ephedrine and adrenaline serves as a better bronchodilator.

b. **Antagonism**: - The phenomenon is referred to as antagonism when one drug's impact is offset or negated by another drug. For e.g., milk of magnesia in acid poisoning.

i. **Chemical antagonism**: - These entail a drug's biological activity being decreased by a chemical reaction with another substance. British anti-Lewisite (dimercaprol; BAL) and arsenic are two examples of acids and alkali. When taking antacids for dyspepsia, sodium bicarbonate must be administered for hydrochloric acid to react with it. Dimerzapam and other chelating drugs are utilised in heavy metal poisoning instances. Deproxamine is administered to treat iron toxicity because it binds sulfhydryl groups to create insoluble complexes that are simple to detoxify.
ii. **Pharmacological antagonism**: There are two categories of antagonists in pharmacology.

(1) **Competitive or reversible antagonism**: This type of antagonism involves competition between the agonist and antagonist for the same receptors. The proportion of receptors that both the chemicals occupy determines how antagonistic the two compounds are. Other characteristics of competitive hostility include:

1. Antagonist and agonist share chemical similarities.

2. By boosting the agonist's concentration at the receptor site, antagonistic effects can be avoided. It implies that the maximum response to the agonist is unaffected.

3. Agonist causes the dosage response curve to move to the right.

4. With a high agonist concentration, the agonist's maximum effect is obtained. The brief duration of action is dependent on medication clearance.

Example: The antagonistic effects of atropine and acetyl choline on muscarinic receptors.

(2) **Non-competitive antagonism**: In this case, the antagonist renders the receptor inactive in a way that prevents the formation of the effective complex with the agonist, regardless of the agonist's concentration. It occurs by any of the following ways:

1. Even at larger concentrations of the agonist, the antagonist may combine at the same location and prevent displacement.

2. In such a case, the antagonist may combine at a different location of the receptor.in which the agonist is fails to start the expected biological reaction

3. The antagonist may cause a specific modification in the receptor by itself, eliminating the reactivity of the receptor spot where the agonist should interact.

Other characteristics of this conflict include:

1. Antagonist differs chemically from agonist.
2. Maximum reaction is muted.
3. The slope of the curve is lessened even if the antagonist moves the dosage response curve to the right.
4. The properties of the antagonist itself determine the magnitude of antagonism, and the agonist has no bearing on either the level of antagonism or its reversibility.
5. Even at high agonist concentrations, Emax of the agonist is lowered.
6. The length of the activity depends on the production of new receptors.

Example: Alpha adrenergic receptors when phenoxybenzamine and adrenaline are combined.

(3) **Physiological antagonism**: Both medications involved in this sort of pharmacological interaction are agonists, which means they each act on a distinct receptor site. They produce opposite actions, which agitate each other's actions.

Example: Histamine and adrenaline. While the latter results in bronchoconstriction, the former causes bronchodilation. In anaphylaxis, adrenalin is a life-saving medication.

15. **Health and Nutrition**: - Weak and anaemic patients are more susceptible to the harmful effects of medication and are therefore given fewer doses. Patients with myxoedema are known to respond less to medicines like amphetamine due to low cellular metabolism, making them more vulnerable to the harmful effects of tetrachloroethylene. Severe anaemia associated with hookworm infection also increases a person's susceptibility to these effects.
16. **Drug dependence**: - Repeated use of drug in an individual leads to production of psychological or physical dependence towards that specific agent. When the dependence is psychological or emotional, it is termed as habituation. E.g., tea, coffee, tobacco, tranquilizers, etc. The withdrawal symptoms of these agents could be easily tackled. On the other hand, if the dependence is physical and psychic, it is termed as addiction. The withdrawal symptoms of some drugs can be fatal and lead to death. So, the drugs which lead to addiction should be prescribed with utter precaution.
17. **Allergy**: - A drug's aberrant response to an antigen-antibody interaction, which releases histamine and histamine-like chemicals, is called an allergy. As a result, there could be bronchoconstriction, urticaria, skin rashes, and a drop in blood pressure. Allergic reactions might happen right once or take many days to manifest. Acute anaphylactic shock brought on by immediate and severe allergic reactions, such as those caused by penicillin, sera,

or vaccinations, can be harmful and even fatal to the patient. In allergic people, penicillin may cause anaphylactic shock (sudden drop in blood pressure), but not in healthy persons. The patient's history of previous allergic responses, the preliminary test dosage, and medications to handle an emergency should therefore be prepared prior to dose calculation.

18. **Idiosyncrasy**: - Due to varied individual susceptibility, the response to every drug varies from person to person. Abnormal or unusual response from the typical pharmacological action of any drug in an individual is termed as idiosyncrasy. For e.g., aspirin may cause gastrointestinal haemorrhage in some patients at even a modest dose, penicillin with sulphonamide can produce certain toxic effects in some individuals.
19. **Tolerance**: - When a drug administered at a standard dose fails to produce the desired pharmacological action, a relatively higher dose of the same is required to exhibit the same response. This distinct resistance hence produced is termed as tolerance, e.g., alcoholics can tolerate larger dose of alcohols, smokers can tolerate nicotine.
20. **Tachyphylaxis**: - It is observed when a drug is administered repeatedly over a short span of time, the receptors get blocked, and the drug's pharmacological effect is reduced ultimately. This cannot be reversed by increasing the dose of the drug. Only if the administration is discontinued for a long time, can the similar effect be observed after future administrations of the same drug. This is termed as tachyphylaxis or acute tolerance. It can be observed with drugs like cocaine, amphetamine, ephedrine, and nitrites.
21. **Metabolic disturbances**: - There is a possibility that the body temperature, water-electrolyte balance, acid-base equilibrium of the body can alter the effect of any medication on it. Salicylates do not possess any antipyretic properties, but they are found to reduce the increased body temperature in patients.

Paediatric Dose Calculations

Accurate dose estimates are crucial in the pharmacy. Every day, pharmacists must calculate both standard and non-standard dosages. A pharmacist is ultimately in charge of all medications and makes the final choice regarding the procedures, equations, and calculations to be applied. Before calculating any dosage, a patient must always consult a registered medical doctor or pharmacist.

Because of their underdeveloped physiological systems, metabolism, weight, and physical condition, children are more vulnerable to drugs than adults. Nurses who give drugs to infants and kids must be watchful to make sure the patient is getting the right medicine. One of the six rights of drug administration—along with the appropriate patient, medication, and route—is the correct dose. time, dosage, and records. The drug will be provided according to the doctor's or provider's prescription. However, the nurse is in charge of making the medication, giving the prescription, and identifying any mistakes in dosage calculation. A tuberculin syringe is required for precise dosing because paediatric dosages are frequently less than 1 mL, as the nurse must be aware of. The kilogramme weight of the infant or child is used to calculate the cost of paediatric drugs. Paediatric doses are typically rounded to the closest tenth. Doses can be adjusted up or down for new-borns and young children. If a youngster weighs more than 50 kg, adult dosages may be administered. Never give a child a dose that is higher than what is advised for an adult. It is always important to keep in mind that many medications have a "do not exceed" or "max. dose" in 24 hours listed. The body surface area (BSA) of the child may also be used by the doctor or pharmacist to determine the amount of medication to be given. When an established dosage has not been set by the pharmaceutical firm, as with some anticancer or specialty medications, the BSA calculation may be utilised.

Most medications are dosed for children based on their body weight (mg/kg) or the surface area of the body (mg/m2), respectively. It is important to accurately convert body weight from pounds to kilogrammes before determining doses based on body weight (1 kg is equivalent to 2.2 lb). Since dosages are frequently specified as mg/kg/day or mg/dose, orders written as "mg/kg/d" are unclear and necessitate further explanation from the prescribing physician. Chemotherapeutic medications are frequently dosed based on body surface area, necessitating a preliminary verification step (BSA calculation). Orders issued in "mL" rather than "mg" are unacceptable since medications come in a variety of concentrations; they need to be clarified. Additionally, dosage varies according to the indication, therefore when determining doses, diagnostic data is useful.

The majority of pharmaceutical reference books concentrate exclusively on adult dosages. However, compared to adults, children may need significantly different pharmaceutical dosages. The correct dosage of medication for a paediatric child can be calculated using a number of different principles, including the Nomogram method, Clark's rule, Fried's rule, and Young's rule.

Now the child's dose is usually calculated from the adult dose according to age, weight, and body surface area by the following methods:

1. **Age**: - When either the manufacturer has not advised dosages for children or the doctor has asked for them to be used, Clark's rule and Young's rule are applied. The fact that children differ so widely in terms of weight, size, tolerances, etc. is the greatest explanation for these. Weight is always expressed in pounds (lbs) rather than kilogrammes (kg) according to Clark's rule.
2. **Young's rule:** - According to this rule, to get a child's drug dosage, multiply the result by the adult dose, divide the result by the child's age, and then add 12 to the child's age.. Thus,

$$\text{Child's dose} = \frac{\text{Age in years}}{\text{Age in years+12}} \text{ x Adult dose}$$

Example: Determine the paediatric dose for a 65-lb girl aged 12 years old. 350 mg is the typical adult dose given for the girl.

Solution: Age of child = 12-year,

Typical adult dose = 350 mg

$$\text{Child's dose} = \frac{\text{Age in years}}{\text{Age in years+12}} \text{ x Adult dose}$$

$$= [12/ (12+ 12)] \text{ x } 350 \text{ mg}$$

$$= (12/24) \text{ x } 350 \text{ mg}$$

$$= 0.5 \text{ x } 350 \text{ mg}$$

$$= 175 \text{ mg}$$

B. **Cowling's rule:** - Children two years of age and older should have their doses calculated according to Cowling's Rule.

$$\text{Child's dose} = \frac{\text{Age at next birthday (in years)}}{\text{Age in years+12}} \text{ x } \underline{\text{Adult}} \text{ dose}$$

C. **Freid's formula** (for infants): - For estimating doses for infants under one year old, use Fried's Rule. By dividing the child's age (in months) by 150 lbs., this rule provides a means to determine the appropriate dosage of medication for a child. The dosage for adults is doubled by the outcome.

$$\text{Child's dose} = \frac{\text{Age in months}}{150} \text{x } \underline{\text{Adult}} \text{ dose}$$

Example: If the recommended dosage for an adult is 500 mg, determine the dose for a 1 year old baby.
Solution: Age of child = 12 months,
Typicaladult dose = 400 mg

$$\text{Child's dose} = \frac{\text{Age in months}}{150} \text{x } \underline{\text{Adult}} \text{ dose}$$

$$= (12/150 \text{ lbs}) \text{ x } 450 \text{ mg}$$
$$= 36 \text{ mg}$$

2. **Body Weight**: - - In order to more correctly dosage medications, doctors frequently prescribe them depending on an adult's or child's body weight. The calculation is quite straightforward and simple to complete. You must pay special attention to whether the dosage is listed in kg or pounds, though. The recommended medicine dosages are deemed appropriate for people weighing 70 kg (150 pounds). The medication concentration at the site of action is influenced by the relationship between the dosage supplied and body mass. Therefore, for individuals who are excessively slim or obese, medicine dosage may need to be changed from the standard adult dose. It is more accurate to calculate a child's medicine dosage based on body weight rather than age.
3. **Clark's rule:** - Although Clark's Rule is an outdated guideline for estimating a child's dosage, paediatric nursing instructors still recommend it for dosage calculations. It is possible to determine the approximate dosage of medication that is appropriate for a child two years of age or older by multiplying the child's weight in pounds by

150 and then dividing the result by the adult dose.

$$\text{Child's dose} = \frac{\text{Weight in pounds}}{\text{150 (average weight of adult in lbs)}} \text{x Adult dose}$$

3. **Body Surface Area**: - Since the proper dosage of medications appears to be more proportionate to surface area, many doctors believe that doses for children should be based on body surface area (BSA). However, there is a close relationship between BSA and a significant number of physiological processes. The BSA is inversely correlated with a number of physiological variables, including plasma volume, oxygen utilisation, and body electrolyte. When administering an anticancer medicine like methotrexate, the dosage is calculated using the BSA at mg/sq. meter of body surface. A 70 kg adult has a BSA of 17 to 18 sq. meter. The given formula is used to calculate the dose for a child depending on BSA:

$$\text{Approximate Child's dose} = \frac{\text{BSA of child (sq.meter)}}{\text{1.8 sq.meter (average adult BSA)}} \text{x Adult dose}$$

A. **Nomogram Method**: The Nomogram method is employed to identify the proper

dose for children's medications dependent on BSA. It accounts for the body surface area of the subject, which for an adult is 1.73 square metres on average (weighing 150-154 lbs). The Nomogram method is the best way because it is based on the patient's height and weight.

$$\text{Child's dose} = \frac{\text{Adult dose}}{1.73} \text{ x Child's BSA}$$

Converting Pounds to Kilograms

To precisely determine prescription dosages and daily fluid requirements for infants and young children, the weight in pounds must be translated to kilogrammes using the formula: **2.2 lbs = 1 kg**. Drug dosages that are safe and effective (S&T) have been determined using kilogramme weights. Always tenths of a kilogramme, never a whole amount, should be used to round the weight.

Example: Determine the dosage for the suspension of amoxycillin (millilitres) for otitis media in a 1-year-old having 26 pounds weight. The dosage is 50 mg/kg/day, divided as needed (b.i.d.). The suspension has a 500 mg/5 mL concentration.

Solution:

1 Convert pounds to kilogrammes: 26 lbs x 1kg/2.2lbs = 11.8 kg

2. Calculate the dosage in mg as follows: 10kg x 50mg/kg/day = 500mg/day

3. Divide the dose by frequency: 500 mg/day ÷ 2 (b.i.d.) = 250 mg/dose (b.i.d.)

4. Converting mg to mL: 250 mg/dose ÷ 500 mg/5 mL = 2.5 mL b.i.d.

Example: Determine the ceftriaxone dosage (millilitres) for a 6-year-old patient weighing 20kg who has meningitis. The dosage is 200 mg/kg/day administered intravenously once daily. The medication has a 50 mg/mL concentration.

Solution:

1. Dosage in mg should be determined as follows: 20kg x 200 mg/kg/day = 4000 mg/day

2. Dose divided by frequency: 4000 mg/day ÷ 1 (daily) = 4000 mg/day

3: Convert mg to mL: 4000 mg/dose ÷ 50 mg/ml = 80 mL once daily

CHAPTER V

Pharmaceutical Calculations

The study of pharmaceutical calculations applies the fundamental ideas of mathematics to the manufacturing and secure and efficient usage of medications. The pharmaceutical calculations are included in the scope of following features:

- the biological activity and rates of drug absorption, body distribution, metabolism, and excretion (pharmacokinetics); and the chemical and physical characteristics of pharmacological compounds and pharmaceutical components.
- statistical information from fundamental investigations and medical drug trials;
- formulation and development of medicinal products;
- Prescriptions and medicine orders, including patient information, drug dose, and dosage schedules compliance;pharmaceutical economics and other things.

Weights & Measures

The standards of weight and measures legislation, which is in place in India, regulates weight and measurement, and the pharmacopoeia has also acknowledged the metric system. The reference standard, secondary standard and working standards are outlined in the Standards of Weights and Measures Act of 1976.

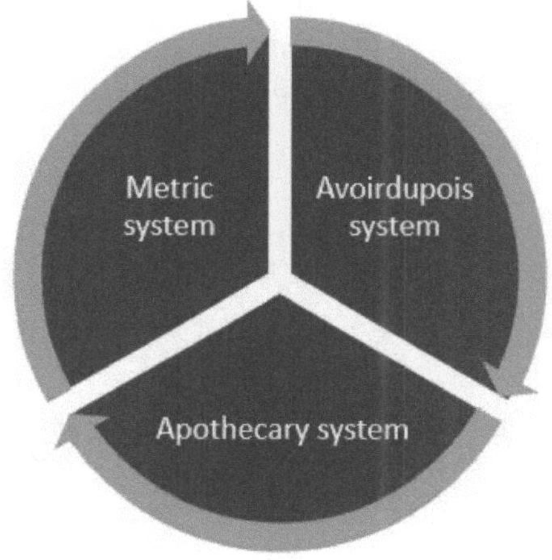

Fig:1.1 Systems of Weights & Measures

PROOF SPIRIT

For a long time, the metric system, the avoirdupois system, and the apothecary system were the three weights and measures used in pharmacies. Despite being written in the avoirdupois or apothecary systems, the pharmacist must translate these prescriptions into the metric system. The metric equivalents specified in the weights and measures (equivalent for dealing with pharmaceuticals) Regulations 1970 (5.1. 1970 No. 1897) must be used when converting prescriptions from older systems. The British Pharmaceutical Codex 1973's Appendix 32 provides information on weights and measures.

THE IMPERIAL SYSTEM

One of the English unit systems is the *Imperial system*. The majority of the units had definitions in many systems, and some of the subsidiary units were employed more extensively or for different reasons in one area than another.

The *Weights and Measures Act* of 1824 and 1878 specified the imperial system of measurement, sometimes known as the British imperial system, as the system of measuring used in the United Kingdom. These include measurements like inches, pounds, gallons, and other units that were widely used in Britain. In this essay, let's study more about the imperial system.

A. **Apothecary System**

When prescribing and dispensing pharmaceuticals in the past, pharmacists and doctors frequently used this system as the system of weights and measures. The less complicated metric system has mostly taken its place, although the pharmacist still runs into these symbols in daily practise. The apothecary system of measurement is still widely employed in a wide range of goods, including pharmaceutical and non-pharmaceutical items.

A. **Avoirdupois System**

The Avoirdupois system is solely a method for measuring weight. Its fundamental unit is the same as the apothecary system's grain. The Avoirdupois ounce and pound are not the same as those used in the apothecary system in terms of way and symbols. Additionally, it is the weight measure used for the purchase and sale of hazardous compounds and over-the-counter medications.

This is crucial to distinguish from the weights used in pharmacy systems, which are only used when a prescription or drug order is placed.

The following is a list of conversions between the prevalent length units used in the Imperial system. :

12 In = 1ft

3 ft = 1 Yard

1760 Yards = 1 mile

Both the metric and the imperial systems of measurement can be used with the time units. Below is a list of conversions between the popular time units:

60 Sec = 1 min

24 hrs = 1day

7days = 1 week

52 weeks = 1 year

<u>IMPERIAL SYSTEM UNITS</u>

Using a few specific units, we can measure length, weight, distance, height, and volume using the imperial system of measurement.

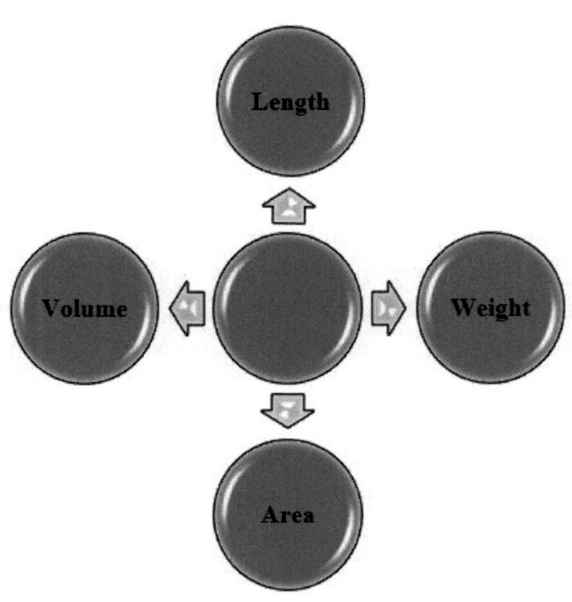

Fig 1.1: Various Measurements

Now , Let's take look in the below table for various imperial system units.
Measurements

Measurements	Units
Length	Inches (in) Feet (ft) Yard (yd) Mile (mi)
Mass / Weight	Grain (gr) Ounce (oz) Quarter (qr or qtr) Stone (st) Pound (lb) Ton (t)
Volume	Fluid ounce (fl oz) Gill (gi) Pint (pt) Quart (qt) Gallon (gal)
Area	Acre Square miles Square feet Square inches

IMPERIAL SYSTEM CHART

You can understand how to convert imperial system units to other imperial units by using the imperial system chart.

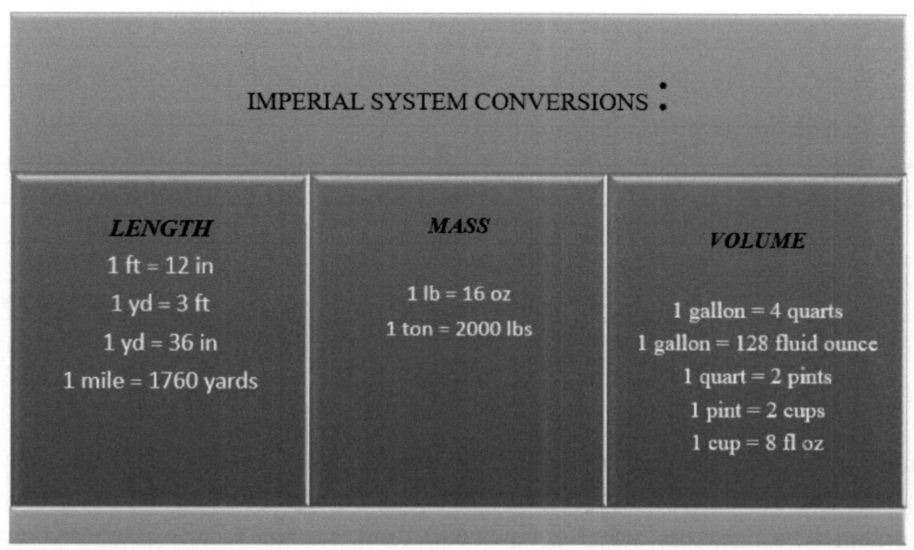

Enter Caption

IMPERIAL SYSTEM EXAMPLES

Example 1: Convert 24 inches to feet.

Solution: The imperial system of measurement uses inches and feet as the units of length measurement. In 1 foot, there are 12 inches. Therefore, there is 1/12 foot in 1 inch.

24 inches = 24 x 1/12 feet = 2 feet

Example 2: Helen determined that a shopping bag weighed 3 kilos, but she needs to know how many pounds that is. Could you assist her with the conversion?

Solution : we must change a unit from the metric system to the imperial system (kg to pounds). One kilogramme weighs about 2.2 pounds.

; 3 kgs = 3 + 2.

THE METRIC SYSTEM

Example 1: Convert 24 inches to feet.

Solution: The imperial system of measurement uses inches and feet as the units of length measurement. In 1 foot, there are 12 inches. Therefore, there is 1/12 foot in 1 inch.

24 inches = 24 x 1/12 feet = 2 feet

The weights and measures (metric system) act was passed in 1897 which legalised the use of the metric system of weights and measures in the nation. In India in 1956, the United States in 1866, and Great Britain in 1864, metric weights were formally acknowledged.

This system's main strengths are its brevity, simplicity, and flexibility to common requirements. Every unit is multiplied or divided by the same number (i.e., 10) to generate different denominations because it is a decimal progression system. Greek prefixes such as deca, hecto, and myria are used to represent multiples of the basic units, while Latin prefixes such as milli, centi, deci, etc. are used to indicate subdivisions.

The metric system's many units are related to one another through the use of

refixes with distinct integer values for each one. Prefixes and their numerical values (written in various ways) include some of the following.

Below is a list of the more popular prefixes along with their numerical values:

CONVERSION TABLE : HIGHER TO LOWER

PREFIX	CONVENTIONAL	DECIMAL
Kilo	1000	-
hecto	100	-
Deka	10	-
Deci	1/10	0.1
Centi	1/100	0.01
Milli	1/1000	0.001
Micro	1/1000,000	0.000001
Nano	1/1000,000,000	0.000000001
pico	1/1000,000,000,000	0.000000000001

LENGTH

Metric length units such the meter, centimeter, millimeter, and smaller are frequently employed in the pharmaceutical industry. The decimeter is hardly ever employed, though. The non-SI term micron is frequently used to refer to the micrometer. The angstrom, which is equal to 0.1 nm, has historically competed with the nanometer in some areas of chemistry.

Using the base units for length:

1 nanometer (nm) =1 m / 100,000,000 = 0,000 000 001 m

1 micrometer (pm) =1 m /1000,000 =0.000001 m
1 millimeter (mm) =1 m / 1000 = 0.001 m
1 centimeter (cm) = 1 m /100 = 0.01 m
1 decimeter (dm) = 1 m / 10 = 0.1 m
1decameter (dam) = 1 m * 10 = 10 m
1 hectometer (hm) =1 m * 100 = 100 m
1 kilometer (km) =1 m * 1000 = 1000 m
1 megameter (Mm) 1 m * 1,000,000 = 1,000,000 m
1 gigameter (Gm) = 1 m * 1,000,000,000 = 1,000,000,000 m

WEIGHT

The metric system uses gram as its base unit of weight. It is equal to the weight of a water ice cube at 4 degree Celcius.

- 1 kilogram (kg) = 1000 grams
- 1 hectagram (hg) = 100 grams
- 1 dekagram (dg) = 10 grams
- 1 gram (g) = 1gram
- 1 decigram (dg) = 0.1 gram
- 1 centigram (cg) = 0.01 gram
- 1 milligram (cg) = 0.001 gram
- 1 microgram (mcg) = 0.000001 gram
- 1 nanogram (ng) = 0.000000001 gram
- 1 picogram (mcg) = 0.000000000001 gram

VOLUME

In Europe, the litre, millilitre, microlitre, and smaller are the most widely used metric units for volume; the centilitre and decilitre are less frequently used for packaged goods.

The units used to describe larger volumes are often kilolitres, megalitres, or gigalitres, or cubic metres.

MEASUREMENT OF CAPACITY

IN METRIC SYSTEM

The volume occupied by a cube with sides of one decimeter is now referred to as a litre (1). The definition of the litre from 1901 has been repealed because a later experiment determined that it to be 1.000028 dm'. The word "litre" is still used in medicine even though it is no longer used to describe the outcomes of very precise volume measurements.

1 Liter (lt) = 1000 milliliters (ml)

CAPACITY MEASURES

1000 ml	1 Quart
500ml	1 pint
30 ml	1 fluid ounce
4 ml	1 fluid drachm
1 ml	15 minim
0.06 ml	1 minim

CONVERSION TABLE FOR DOMESTIC MEASURES

DOMESTIC MEASURE	METRIC SYSTEM	IMPERIAL SYSTEM
1 drop	0.06 ml	1 minim
1 tea spoonful	4.00 ml	1 fluid drachm
1 desert spoonful	8.00 ml	2 fluid drachm
1 table spoonful	15.00 ml	4 fluid drachm
2 table spoonful	30.00 ml	1 fluid ounce
1 wine glassful	60.00 ml	2 fluid ounce
1 tumblerful	240.00 ml	8 fluid ounce

CALCULATIONS BASED ON DENSITY:

The mass of a substance per unit volume is the idea of density. It uses mass units rather than volume units.

The mass of a substance in air divided by the mass of the same amount of water is known as specific gravity.Both density and specific gravity are quantitatively identical in the metric system.

DENSITY = WEIGHT / VOLUME

EXAMPLE :

The density of pure glycerin is 1,25g/ml then calculate the volume of 2kg of glycerin.

SOLUTION :

As we know ,

VOLUME = WEIGHT / DENSITY
= 2000 g / 1.25 g/ml
= 1600 ml

Therefore , the volume of glycerin was found to be 1600m

IMPERIAL SYSTEM v/s METRIC SYSTEM

Some nations employ the imperial system, while others rely on the metric system. We must comprehend the distinction between the metric and imperial measurement systems. To compare the imperial and metric systems, see the table below.

Imperial system Vs Metric system

Imperial system	Metric system
The imperial system is the name for the measurement system used in countries like the UK, Liberia, Myanmar, etc. that uses units like an inch, pound, tonne, etc..	A decimal system of units based on metres, kilogrammes, and seconds as the appropriate units of length, mass, and time is known as the metric system. These are the "Systeme International" units, or SI units.
The conversion units don't comply to any particular pattern. There are 12 inches in a foot, three feet in a yard, etc.	As units are based on powers of 10, it is based on the decimal system. For instance, 1 mile = 1000 metres, 1 litre =1000 millilitres, etc.
Imperial system units includes,: Inches, Yard, Foot, Mile, Pound, Ounce, Gallon, etc.	Whereas Metric system units include : Meter, Centimeter, Liter, Kiloliter, Gram, Kilogram, millimeter, etc.

Let us read the chart given below showing the metric system to imperial system conversions.

Metric Units

Metric Units	Imperial Units
1 Centimeter	0.394 Inch
1 Meter	3.281 Feet or 1.093 yards
1 Kilometer	0.621 mile
1 Gram	0.035 ounce
1 Kilogram	2.205 pounds
1 Litre	0.034 fluid ounce
1 Mililitre	1.057 quart or 0.264 gallon

PERCENTAGE SOLUTIONS

The advent of the metric system has made many calculations required in the practise of pharmacy simpler, particularly those involving the quantities required to generate percentage solutions. The percentage of a solute in the solvent is one way to express the concentration of a solution.

The British Pharmacopoeia defines 4 different types of percentage solutions, :

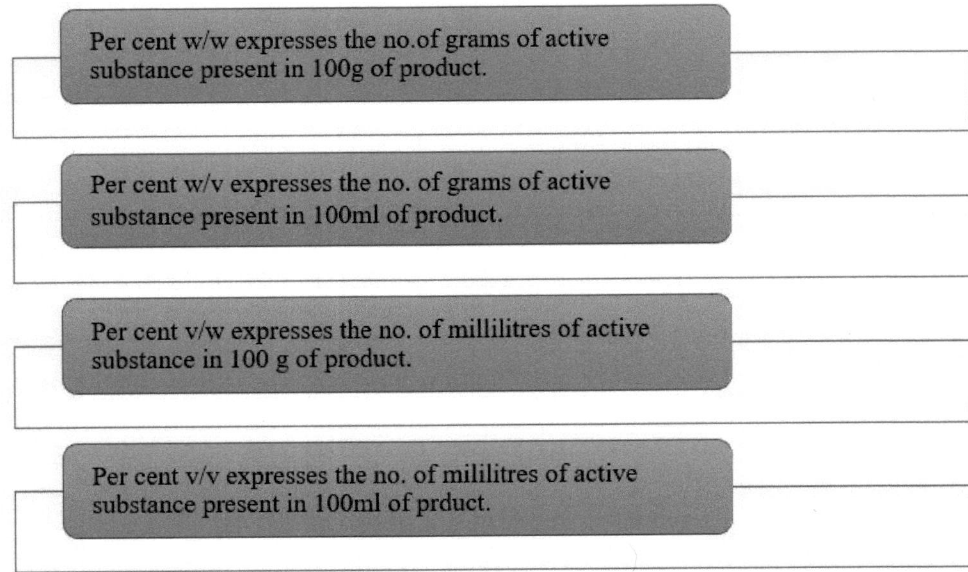

It needs to be noted that when calculating percent w/v solutions, the solvent's density is not taken into consideration. Thus, 5 g of phenol are present in 100 ml of water in a 5 per Cent w/v solution of phenol in water. Similar to this, 5g phenol is present in a 5 percent w/v solution in glycerin that includes enough glycerin to make 100 ml of solution.

<u>Conversion of Percentage Strength to Millimoles Per Litre</u>

Let C percentage w/v strength of salt

W = milligrams of salt containing 1 millimole of the specified ion

100 mililitres of solution contain C grams of salt , 1 litre of solution contains 10* C grams of salt = 10,000 C milligrams

Therefore,

Milimoles per litre = 10,000 C/ W

The percentage strength of a salt that contains the given ion can be used to determine the number of millimoles per litre using this equation.

Example 1:

How many millimoles per litre of bicarbonate ion are contained in a solution of sodium bicarbonate 8.4 per cent w/v?

Solution : C= 8.4 per cent w/v

W = 84 milligrams

Therefore, Milimoles per litre = 10,000*8.4 /84

= 1000

Ans. 8.4 w/v solution of sodium bicarbonate contains 1000 millimoles of bicarbonate per litre.

PERCENT BY WEIGHT

The weight of the solute divided by the total weight of the solution, multiplied by 100%, is the definition of percent by mass (w/w).

% w/w = <u>Weight of solute</u> * 100%

Total weight of solution

Example 1: What is the %w/w of a solution that contains 20 g of lactose in 400 g of solution?

Solution: Percent by mass = <u>Mass of lactose</u> * 100%

Total mass of solution

= 20 g / 400 g x 100%

= 5 % w/w

PERCENT BY VOLUME

The term percent by volume (v/v) is defined as the volume of the solute divided by the total volume of the solution multiplied by 100%.

% w/v = Volume of solute * 100%

Total volume of solution

Example 1: How would you prepare 300 ml of 60 % (v/v) of rubbing alcohol?

Solution:

60% = Volume of rubbing alcohol *100 %

Total volume of solution

Volume ofRubbing alcohol = 60% * 300 ml

100%

= 180 ml

Therefore , you would add enough water to 180 ml of rubbing alcohol to make a total of 300 ml of the solution

Other ways to indicate solution percentages include w/v and v/v in addition to w/v and v/v. Concentration can also be expressed in different ways.

The most common way to express a solution's concentration is by its molarity. a few formulae for temperature-dependent concentration. As the temperature varies, the solution's concentration alters.

MOLARITY :

The number of moles of a solute contained in exactly one litre of a solution is known as molarity. The capital "M" is used to denote it. To calculate the molarity of a solute in solution, we need to know both the number of moles of a solute present in the solution and the volume of the solution (in litres). Equation used to determine molarity of a solution expressed as :

Molarity (M) = Moles of solute

Volume of Solution in litres

MOLALITY :

The number of moles of solute that are dissolved in exactly one kilograms (1000 grams) of solvent is known as the molality (m). Keep in mind that the word "molality" is spelled with two Ts and is represented by a lowercase "m."

To determine the molality of a solute in a solution, we need to know the moles of solute present in the solution and the mass of solvent (in kilogrammes) in the solution. The following equation is used to determine molality:

Molality (m) = moles of solute

Volume of solvent in kilograms

MOLE FRACTION :

The mole fraction (X) of a component in a solution is the proportion of that component's moles to the total moles of all the other components in the solution.We need to know how many moles of each component are present in the solution in order to determine the mole fraction. The following equation is used to get the mole fraction of component A. X in a mixture of components A, B, and C:

X_A = Moles of A

Moles of A + Moles of B

\+ Moles of C

X_B : Moles of B

Moles of A + Moles of B

\+ Moles of C

ALLIGATION METHOD

The word "alligation," which derives from the Latin "alligatio," which meaning "the art of attaching," refers to the lines that are formed during calculations to connect different quantities. Alligation is a simple arithmetical method for determining the ratio in which solutions or other substances of various percentage strengths should be combined to create a mixture after mixing solutions or other substances having various concentrations of active ingredients.

This technique involves calculating the strength of a mixture of more than two substances with known strengths. There are 2 types of alligation methods.

Alligation medial :

The main purpose of medial alligation is to determine the quantity of a mixture from the quantities of its constituent parts. In other words, this method is used to determine how much of an active component is present in each substance that makes up a compound as well as how much of an active ingredient is there overall. Whether they are expressed in weight or volume, the quantities are given in a standard denomination.

EXAMPLE : 1

In a mixture of 3000 ml of 40% v/v alcohol, 1000 ml of 60% v/v alcohol, and 1000 ml of 70% v/v alcohol, what is the percentage strength of alcohol (v/v)? After mixing, assume no volume contraction. (What per cent of 5000 is 2500 ?)

Solution : 0.4 × 3000 mL = 1200, or 40% alcohol in 3000 ml

0.6 x 1000 mL = 600, or 60% alcohol in 1000 ml

0.7 x 1000 ml = 700, or 70% alcohol in 1000 mL

Totals: 3000+ 1000+ 1000 = 5000 mL (total amount of alcoholic solution)

1200+ 600+ 700 = 2500 mL (total amount of alcohol in solution)

Therefore, 2500 mL/5000 mL = 0.5 x 100 = 50%

Thus, 50% is the strength (v/v) of alcohol present in a mixture of 5000 mL

ALLIGATION ALTERNATE :

Alligation alternate is defined as a method used to find the amount of each ingredient needed make a mixture of a given quantity. A mixture's strength must fall somewhere between that of its constituent parts; specifically, it must be both somewhat stronger than its weakest component and slightly weaker than its strongest component . Alternate alignment is more difficult and requires arranging the materials.involve into high and low pairs which are then traded-off.

PROOF SPIRIT

It is an alcoholic drink with a standard percentage of alcohol in it, or an alcohol and water mixture. With a specific gravity of 0.91976 at 15.5°C and a concentration of 57.1% v/v or 49.28% w/w ethyl alcohol, the proof spirit is typically described in Great Britain as a mixture of absolute alcohol and water that weighs exactly 12/13 equal volumes of water at 51°F.

The term "proof spirit" refers to any alcoholic solution that is 100 proof and includes 57.1% V/V alcohol. Alcoholic preparations' strengths are described as "over proof" (O.P.) or "under proof" degrees for excise purposes (U.P.). Any strength above proof strength is expressed as over proof (O.P.) and any strength below proof strength is expressed as under proof (U.P.).

Any % V/V of alcohol can be converted into proof strength and vice versa:

57.1 volumes of ethyl alcohol = 100 volume of proof spirit

Therfore, 1 volume of ethyl alcohol =100/57.1

i.e, 1.753 volumes of proof spirit

Aqueous solutions holding 50% by volume of absolute alcohol (100 percent ethanol) are known as proof spirits. The proof strength is double the alcohol strength in percentage terms, 50% v/v alcohol equals 100 proofs. Reversed, 45% v/v ethanol is the same as 90 proofs of alcohol. A proof gallon of alcohol can be purchased for manufacturing purposes. A proof gallon is a gallon of proof spirit, or 100 proof or 50% v/v absolute alcohol, by measure.

ISOTONIC SOLUTIONS

EXAMPLE 1 : A sample of brandy is 40 under proof . Calculate its alcoholic strength v/v ?

Solution :

40 under proof = 40-100 = 60

Alcoholic strength = 60/ 1.753 = 34.2 % v/v

- Isotonic solutions are which have same osmotic pressure or equal solute concentrations.
- a solution with the same quantity of salt in it as blood and cells. Isotonic solutions are often used as intravenous fluids in hospitalised patients.
- Since 0.9% sodium chloride solution is thought to pass the same osmotic pressure as blood plasma, it is a standard solution..
- **Any concentration above this (0.9%) is considered as hypertonic and below this (0.9%) is considered as hypotonic.**
- Isotonic describes medicinal dose formulations that are compatible with bodily fluids. Saline solutions, for instance, are isotonic with both blood and lachrymal fluid. When the formulation is isotonic with bodily fluids, administration doesn't result in any annoyance or discomfort.

ADJUSTMENT OF TONICITY

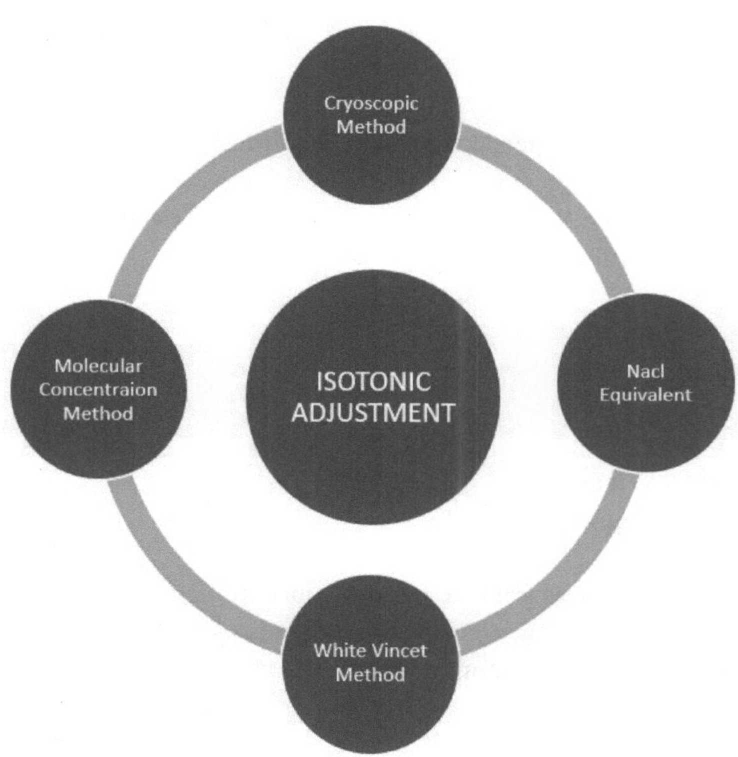

1. **Freezing Point Method / Cryoscopic Method**

The FP of the lachrymal fluid is 0.52°C and it contains solutes. all potential solutions. which are isotonic with the lachrymal fluid and freeze at -0.52°C. Similar to how human blood plasma does, any solutions with FP at -0.52°C will be isotonic with blood plasma.

A method for calculating a substance's molecular weight by dissolving it and measuring its freezing point.

% w/v of adjusting substance needed = $\frac{0.52 - PSM * a}{b}$

Where,

PSM stands for = percentage strength of medicament

a= FP of unadjusted solution

b= FP of a 1% w/v solution of adjusting substance

EXAMPLE:

How to manufacture a 1% solution of blood plasma-based iso osmotic boric acid. [Hint: Boric acid solution at 1% w/v has a FP of 0.2880 c. The freezing point of a sodium chloride solution at 1% w/v is 0.576 °C.]

SOLUTION :

Percentage of w/v of sodium chloride = 0.52 –PSM * a

b

= 0.52 – 1 * 0.288

0.576

= 0.402% w/v

Therefore , 0.402 g of Nacl requires 1 g of boric acid to become isotonic..

2. **NACL EQUIVALENT METHOD :**

Quantity of NaCl required to adjust tonicity = 0.9 – (PSM * E)

Where ,

PSM = % strength of medicament

E = Nacl equivalent (the amount of nacl needed to make 1 g of drug)

3. WHITE VINCET METHOD :

The White–Vincent method uses the NaCl equivalent value of the material By multiplying the material's mass and its NaCl equivalent value by 111.1 as a constant, to obtain isotonic solution.

V = W * E * 111.1

Where ,

V = volume of isotonic solution in ml

W = drug weight

E = equivalent of Nacl

4. MOLECULAR CONCENTRATION

% W/V of adjusting substance required = 0.03 M

N

Molar concentration is a unit of measurement for the concentration of a chemical species, particularly the concentration of a solute in a solution. As the freezing point decreases the solute concentration increases. In other words, it depends on the number of ions (or, more precisely, the number of effective ions), the weight of the drug, and the molecular weight of the substance.

Where ,

M = gram molecular weight

N = no. of ions

EXAMPLE:

How we can prepare a dextrose-based iso osmotic solution?

HINT: Dextrose's molecular weight is 180.

SOLUTION :

Dextrose is non ionizing substance

W = 0.03 M

Therefore ,

W = 0.03 * 180 = 5.4g / 100ml

MODEL QUESTIONS

1. Discuss various ways to express solution strengths.
2. What is percentage solutions ?
3. Calculate proof strength of 55% v/v and 45 % v/v alcohol

4. Classify systems of measurements

CHAPTER VI

POWDERS

LEARNING OBJECTIVES

The following are some of the chapter's goals:

- to comprehend the idea of powder and become familiar with its classification, benefits, and drawbacks.
- to become familiar with the many varieties of granules and powders.
- To familiarise oneself with the general formulations' techniques and guiding principles. in the study and development of formulations, to comprehend the physical properties of powders and granules.
- Classification of powders
- advantages and disadvantages of powders
- Simple and compound powders – their official preparations, dusting powders, effervescent and efflorescent and hygroscopic powders,
- eutectic mixtures and Geometric dilutions.

INTRODUCTION

Pharmaceutical powder are solid dosage forms for medications that contain more than one medicines that are dispersed in a very finely divided condition, with excipients or without excipients. They come in amorphous or crystalline forms.

- Historically, powders represent one of the' oldest dosage forms.
- Using powder as a dose form enables medications to be broken down into a very fine state, which frequently increases their therapeutic activity or efficacy by speeding up the rate of dissolution and/or absorption.
- To manufacture ointments, pastes, suppositories, and other products, powdered medications are routinely combined with other ingredients.
- Despite the fact that medicines are being manufactured in a variety of distinct physical forms, the most of them are made utilising powders of some sort or another.

ADVANTAGES OF POWDERS:

Each dosage form produced in this manner has some benefits over the others. Similar to that, the powders provide the following benefits:

i. the majority of medications are offered in powder form, making it more , It is practical for the physician to prescribe a certain dosage of medication.in accordance with the patient's needs.
v. Powders' smaller particle size results in a more rapid dissolution compared to other solid dosage forms of medication, like pills, tablets or capsules.
v. The action is generated in a less amount of time due to the quick dissolution, which increases blood concentration in a shorter amount of time.
v. They are more easy to carry as compared to liquid dosage forms.
v. Powders are usually more stable than liquids as the rate of chemical decomposition reaction is higher in case of liquids dosage forms in atmospheric conditions.
v. The easiest way to administer medications that must be taken in big doses is to mix them with food or beverages in powder form.
v. Powders have a small particle size, large surface area, & are rapidly digested in the digestive tract, which minimises the issues with local irritation.

DISADVANTAGES OF POWDERS:

Bulk powders should not be used to administer potent medications in low doses.

v. Unsuitable for medications that are unstable in a typical atmosphere.
v. Bitter , nauseous ,and unpalatable medicaments cannot be dispersed in powdered form.
v. Deliquescent and hygroscopic medications are packaged in double wrapping because they cannot be administered in powder form.
v. Volatile drugs cannot be dispensed in powdered form.
v. Powders are vulnerable to physiological instability.
v. Inconvenient to carry

CLASSIFICATION OF POWDERS:

Although tablets and capsules have mostly overtaken powders as a dose form in modern medicine, powders nevertheless rank among the earliest and still have several benefits that make them useful for pharmaceutical dosage forms.

Powders can be classified in various types :

1. **Powders for internal use includes**

A. Divided Powders

- Simple
- Compound
- Powders Enclosed in Cachets
- Tablet Triturates

A. **Powders for external use includes**
B. Dusting Powders

- Medicated dusting powder
- Surgical dusting powder

B. Insufflations
C. Douche Powder
D. Dentrifices

3. **Special Powders includes**

A. Eutectic Mixture
B. Effervescent Powder

POWDERS FOR INTERNAL USE

Oral powders are characterised as finely milled powders that contain one or more drugs, either with or without auxiliary substances, including, various indicated, flavoring and coloring additives, by Indian Pharmacopoeia 2007.

With or without the aid of water or any other suitable liquid, they are meant to be consumed internally.

A. Divided Powder:

Single dosages of powdered drugs, commonly referred to as divided powders or charta, are individually wrapped in paper, foil, or cellophane. Split powder is a more accurate dosage form than bulk powder because the patient is not involved in the dosage measurement procedure. Divided powders are sold commercially in foil, cellophane, or paper.

SIMPLE POWDER:

- Each individual dose is packed in paper in this powder form. There may be just one (basic) ingredient or several (compound)
- Simple powders are made up of just one ingredient and can be crystalline or amorphous; when it is crystalline, it is reduced to a fine powder.
- Each powder should be present in a minimum of 100 mg.
- Example : Dispense six powders of aspirin each powder contains 300mg of aspirin.

Rx

Aspirin 300mg Make a powder

Direction: One powder should be taken after every eight hours

Method: Weigh the needed amount of aspirin after powdering the aspirin. For each powder, weigh 300 milligrams of aspirin. Wrap each dose in a separate piece of powder paper. Make six of these powders. Wrap it up from flap to flap and secure with an elastic band.

COMPOUND POWDER

These type of powders category contains more than two substances which are mixed together and then divided into individual doses.

EXAMPLE : Dispense eight powders of A.P.C

Rx

Aspirin 300mg

Paracetamol 150mg

Caffeine 50mg

Direction : When need arises one powder should be taken

Procedure: Weigh the calculated amount of each component after powdering all the ingredients. In descending order of weight, combine them. For each powder, weigh 500mg of the combined powder. Wrap each dose in a separate piece of powder paper. Pack with elastic band restrained in pairs, flap to flap.

POWDERS ENCLOSED IN CACHETS:

- The solid unit dose form of medication known as a cachet is difficult to swallow as a whole but simple to prepare and dissolves quickly in the stomach.
- The contents of a cachet are a dry powder contained in a shell that is typically made by moulding a mixture of rice flour and water into the desired form and drying it.
- They can contain a larger dose than a tablet or capsule and are very helpful for giving medications with nauseous and unpleasant tastes.
- A capsule has mostly supplanted a cachet because it provides less protection against light and moisture.

TYPES OF CACHETS:

There are 2 types of cachets

A. Wet seal &

B. Dry seal cachets

Wet seal cachets:

Two comparable convex sections with flat edges together create a wet seal cachet. One half, the edges of which are moistened with water, is then fitted precisely over the first half containing the medication and the measured amount of powdered medication is placed within.

?DIRECTION FOR USE : IMMERSE IT IN THE WATER FOR FEW SECONDS AND THEN SWALLOW IT WITH DRAUGHT OF THE WATER.

DRY SEAL CACHETS

Dry seal cachets contains two halves, the upper & the lower half, with the upper half having a somewhat greater diameter. The lower half of the powdered medicine is filled, and the upper half is fitted over the lower half. The two pieces are then pushed together to mechanically seal the filled cachets. The cachets are taken out of the filling and placed in boxes.

The powder cannot leak from the dry seal cachets, which may be made more efficiently and with greater hygienic standards.

Example include , Sodium Amino salicylate Cachets ,

Sodium Amino salicylate with Isoniazid Cachets.

DISPENSING OF CACHETS

The cachets are placed in tins or boxes, either laying flat or piled on their edges. The compartments may be filled with cotton wool if necessary. The following instructions should be included on the label of cachets: "Immerse in water for a few seconds and then swallow with a draught of water."

TABLET TRITURATES

- These are tablets made of powder. Molded tablets are circular, flat discs that typically contain a powerful drug diluted with lactose, dextrose, or another appropriate diluent.
- The equipment used to prepare tablet triturates is comprised of plastic or stainless steel.
- It consists of an upper perforated plate with precisely the same number of holes as the lower plate's lower plate's number of pegs. Two additional big pegs on the lower plates assure proper plate alignment.
- When the top plate is lightly pressed, it will glide lower and leave the moulded tablets on the protruding pegs. The tablets are spread out in single layers on a clean surface and dried either by keeping them in a warm area or using a hot air oven.
- Presently, automatic tablet triturators, including tablet makers, can also be used to create tablet triturates. 2500 tablet triturates can be produced by a tablet triturate machine every minute.

USES :

- They are used for oral administration or for sublingual use (nitroglycerin tablets,)
- They can be put inside capsules, which solves the issue of accurately estimating the dosage of strong medications in powder form.
- Examples includes : Propranolol Scopolamine Tablet Triturate

POWDERS FOR EXTERNAL USE

A. **DUSTING POWDER**

Bulk powders applied externally are called dusting powders. They are free-flowing, extremely fine powders that contain lubricants, antiseptics, antipruritics , astringents, and antiperspirants. To open wounds, only sterile dusting powders should be used .The typical packaging for dusting powders is glass or metal with a perforated cover.

They are of 2 types :

MEDICATED DUSTING POWDERS

- Medicated dusting powders are used mainly for superficial skin conditions,
- Medicated dusting powders are sterile and intended for use on the surface of the skin. Body dusting powders are popular because to their smooth texture and cooling effect, both of which are caused by the vast surface area of the talc particles, which also contributes to additional heat loss.
- Eczema, Pleurodesis, Skin Irritation, Hemorrhoids, Minor Skin Infections, Nappy Rashes, Sunburn, and other disorders are treated with medicated mentholated dusting powder.

SURGICAL DUSTING POWDERS

- Surgical dusting powders are designed to be applied to serious wounds, such as burns and a baby's umbilical cord, as well as to deep layers of skin.
- Prior to usage, surgical dusting powders must be sterilised to ensure that they are free of pathogenic microorganisms

Dusting powder is mainly used for their antiseptic, astringent, absorbent, and antipruritic action.

Dispense 50g of dusting powders

Rx

- Sterilized purified talc = 50.0g
- Starch in powdered form = 25.0g
- Zinc oxide in powdered form = 20.0g
- Salicylic acid in powdered from = 5.0g
- Make a powder

Method: Weigh the necessary amount of salicylic acid, starch, zinc oxide, and pure talc. In descending order of weight, combine them. Once sifting it once more, lightly stir the powder after it has been blended. To shield it from contamination from the environment, transfer the powder into sifter-top containers.

Example: Ø Neosporin Dusting Powder Ø composed of the following active ingredients (salts)

Ø Bacitracin (5000 IU)

Ø Neomycin (3400 IU)

Ø Polymyxin B (400 IU)

B. INSUFFLATIONS

- Medicated dusting powders known as insufflations are introduced into body cavities like the nose, throat, ears, etc. with the aid of a device called an insufflator (powder blower).
- The powder is sprayed all over the application site in a stream of finely divided particles.
- The particle size of insufflations must be extremely small, and they must be completely free of irritating and sensitising effects.
- The insufflations are used to either generate a local effect from a drug that is broken down in the digestive system, such as when antibiotics are used for treating ear, nose, and throat infections, or to produce a systemic effect from a drug.
- Insufflations may not produce a consistent dose, just as aerosols.
- Examples include powdered Cromolyn sodium and Clioquin powder USP

C. DOUCHE POWDER

Douche powders are primarily used for vaginal use, although they can also be manufactured for nasal, otic, or ophthalmic use. They are designed to be used as antiseptics or cleansing agents for a bodily cavity.

Aromatic oils are frequently used in the manufacturing of douche powder. To avoid agglomeration and to guarantee thorough mixing, it becomes necessary to run them through a sieve of 40 or 60.

They can be administered either in powder boxes or wide mouth glass bottles, however the former is recommended due to the protection provided against air and moisture from environment.

Zinc sulphate, Magnesium sulphate, Boric acid, Lemon oil, and purified water are a few examples of douche powder.

D. DENTRIFICES

These are used to clean the surface of the teeth when using a toothbrush. They include an appropriate amount of detergent or soap, an abrasive material, and an appropriate flavour. Fine powder forms of abrasives such calcium sulphate, magnesium carbonate, sodium carbonate, and sodium chloride are employed.

A powerful abrasive should not be used, though, as it could harm the tooth's structure.

Rx

Hard soap, in fine powdered form = 50.0g

Precipitated calcium carbonate = 935.0g

Saccharin sodium = 2.0g

Peppermint oil = 4.0g

Cinnamon oil = 2.0ml

Methyl salicylate = 8.0ml

Make a tooth powder

EUTECTIC MIXTURE

Eutectic mixtures are substances with low melting points that, when combined, become liquids because the mixture's melting point is lowered below room temperature. They are combinations of materials that melt when combined, rubbed, or triturated. Eutectic substances liquefy to varying degrees depending on their melting points, relative amounts, and ambient temperature. The emergence of eutectic mixtures denotes a physical transformation as opposed to a chemical one.

Menthol, acetanilide, thymol, phenacetin, camphor, aspirin, phenol, antipyrine, salol, and chloral hydrate are the chemicals that liquefy when mixed.

When combined, any two of these medications become liquid. This issue during the manufacture of powders of such materials can be resolved by distributing the individual components of the eutectic mixture individually and employing inert adsorbents like starch, talc, or lactose to prevent the powder from becoming moist.

EFFERVESCENT POWDERS

The ingredients in effervescent powders react with water to produce carbon dioxide. The constituents for this class of treatments can either be compounded as granules or distributed as salts.

The evolution of the gas requires the presence of a soluble carbonate, such as sodium bicarbonate, and an organic acid, such as citric or tartaric acid. The medication can be given in either a bulk powder form or as individual powders..

The saline and bitter taste of medications are covered up by the carbonated water that results from the emission of carbon dioxide, and carbon dioxide is also thought to enhance gastric juice flow and hasten drug absorption.

When introducing compounds to water, effervescent granules are preferred to effervescent powders since they dissolve substances more slowly. Additionally, as if powders are employed, there could be fierce and uncontrollable effervescence and carbon dioxide loss, which could significantly reduce the solution's carbonation

PREPARATION OF POWDER

1. **Particle size reduction :**

When making powder, When manufacturing powder materials, the manufacturer must use a variety of methods and equipment to reduce the particle size.; this is known as comminution. The process of trituration, which involves putting the solid in a mortar and repeatedly applying force downward between the pestle and the mortar to grind the chemical, is the most widely employed for reducing particle size in powder formulation. To make sure that all of the particles are equally reduced and combined, the powder needs to be constantly scraped off the sides of the mortar. The solid can be treated by either continuing the trituration process or by putting the mixture on an ointment slab and applying a levigating ingredient, such as glycerin.

2. **Preparing a homogeneous mixture :**

Preparing a homogeneous mixture: After particle size reduction, all powder ingredients are thoroughly blended together. For obtaining homogeneous mixtures, techniques frequently resembling those used for particle size reduction are employed. Powders that have been appropriately combined under little to no pressure must have a protectant added to them to prevent the formation of a eutectic mixture. Trituration serves the dual purposes of lowering particle size and mixing powders. Spatulation produces a light, well-combined powder without affecting the protectant when particles are blended with a spatula on an ointment slab.. It works particularly well when combining smaller doses of powerful medications with bigger volumes of diluents. Tumbling is a technique that can be used to successfully combine hazardous materials. The powders are placed in transparent bottles with lids or zipper-sealed bags and stirred until thoroughly combined. Adding a colouring ingredient can help determine the mixture's homogeneity. The geometric dilution approach is employed if the quantities of the powders being mixed are not equal.

3. **Geometric dilution :**

By using geometric dilution method , it is possible to combine or distribute two or more substances evenly. When mixing strong chemicals with a lot of diluents, this process is intended.

- The potent medicine is added to a mortar along with nearly equal amounts of diluent, and the mixture is thoroughly mixed by trituration.
- The trituration process is repeated after adding a second part of diluent that is volumetrically equivalent to the powder combination in the mortar.
- Equal amounts of diluents are continuously added to the powder mixture present in the mortar till all of it is contents are integrated.

For example:
If the dosage of a potent medicine is 120 mg, the complete 120 mg dose should be taken, along with 120 mg of diluents, and well mixed. When all of the diluents have been added, the
240 mg powerful drug and diluent mixture is combined once more with another 240 mg of diluents.

4. **Packaging of powders :**

To make topical application easier, Bulk powders for external use (also known as dusting powders) are frequently distributed in shaker-top containers. They can also be administered in a plastic container with a flip-top cover or a wide-mouth jar. For greater stability and defence against light and moisture, the jar or plastic container can be firmly closed, especially for mixtures that contain volatile substances. Labels on the package should state "For external usage only."

Bulk powders meant for internal consumption should be administered in a jar with a tight-fitting lid that is amber in colour and has a large opening. They should come with a dosage spoon or cup that is the right size. The strength of the active component per dose should be listed on the label of bulk powders intended for internal use (e.g., Potassium chloride 600 mg per tablespoonful).

PROBLEMS ENCOUNTERED IN POWDER FORMULATION

1. **EFFLORESCENT POWDERS :**

Due to changes in relative humidity or during trituration, crystalline solids can partially or completely release water from crystallisation, resulting in the powder becoming moist or liquefying. Use of the matching anhydrous salt or the mixing of an inert substance with the efflorescent substance before adding the other ingredients can solve this problem.

Example include caffeine, citric acid, and ferrous sulphate etc.

2. **HYGROSCOPIC POWDERS & DELIQUESCENT POWDER :**

Substances which absorb moisture from the atmosphere are not suitable for dispensing in powder papers because the absorbed moisture may promote the chemical degradation of the drug because the absorbed moisture may promote the chemical degradation of the drug. In the case of effervescent preparations, cause the acids to completely react with the sodium bicarbonate, rendering the preparation useless.

Several precautions to be taken while dispensing such powders are:

- In order to expose less surface area to the atmosphere, the hygroscopic chemicals are often given in granular form.
- Hygroscopic powders shouldn't be ground to a fine powder. In the event that it is necessary, the powdering can be done in a dried and warmed mortar.
- Such powders should be packaged in two layers. It is best to further wrap items in aluminium foil or plastic cover when the weather is humid or while working with particularly liquefiable materials.

Some of the examples include , ammonium chloride, ammonium bromide, ammonium iodide, calcium chloride, hyoscine bydro bromide, iron and ammonium citrate, pepsin, phenobarbitone sodium, potassium citrate, sodium bromide, sodium iodide, citric and tartaric acid.

3. **INCORPORATION OF LIQUIDS :**

Some powders require the addition of liquid substances in addition to the solid elements. It's important to distribute fluids properly throughout the entire powder. In this instance, the powder is first triturated with the liquid in an amount equal to its weight before the remaining powder is added. To prevent this issue, adsorbent is used, such as light kaolin.

4. **INCORPORATION OF EXTRACTS :**

Some plant extracts are offered as semisolids or powders (for example, liquid extract of liquorice). In this situation, powdered extracts behave normally and are treated as powders. Before incorporating semisolid extract with other ingredients, it should be combined with an equivalent amount of lactose and evaporated to a dry powder. If heating is necessary, it must be done carefully to preserve the extract's efficacy.

5. **INCOMPATIBLE SALTS :**

Triturating salts that are chemically incompatible results in colour change, chemical deterioration, or loss of potency. The use of little pressure when compounding such materials helps to avoid this issue. Use a practical mixing technique, such as jar tumbling or spatulation on paper, to combine the powder. The materials should be gently blended after each substance has been ground separately in a clean mortar. These substances are powdered and administered separately if not.

6. **EXPLOSIVE MIXTURE :**

When triturated in a mortar with a reducing agent, such as sulphides, sulphur, tannic acid, and charcaol, oxidising substances such as potassium salts of chlorate, dichromate, permanganate, and nitrate, sodium peroxide, silver nitrate, and silver oxide violently explore when heated at a high temperature. To minimise this problem, each salt is triturated separately, or only mild pressure is used while triturating.

EVALUATION OF POWDER

Pharmaceutical powders are evaluated on the basis of following quality control parameters:

1. **Content uniformity**
2. **Particle size and size distribution**
3. **Flow property :**

(a) Angle of repose
(b) Flow rate

4. **Density**

(a) Bulk density
(b) Tapped density
(c) True density

5. **Hausner's ratio**
6. **Moisture content**
7. **Tensile & Cohesive Strength**
8. **Safety and Efficacy**
9. **Stability**

MODEL QUESTIONS :

1. Define and give example of simple and compound powders
2. Explain the problems encountered in powder formulation ?
3. Write a note on :

A. Eutectic mixtures
B. Efflorescent powder
C. Geometric dilution
D. Give the preparation of dusting and effervescent powders .

CHAPTER VII

Liquid Dosage Forms

Liquid Dosage forms

Oral liquids are homogenous liquid solutions that typically contain one or more active components suspended or emulsified in a suitable liquid foundation. Liquid dosage forms include syrup, oral suspension, oral solution, oral drop, oral emulsion, mixture, linctus, and elixir .

When compared to solid and semisolid dose forms, liquid dosage forms offer many patients unique advantages such as greater dosage management and better patient compliance, especially for individuals who have trouble swallowing. Pharmacy uses a variety of liquid dose forms. Depending on the type of medicine, its solubility, and its stability, liquid dosage forms are created as either solutions, suspensions, or emulsions. Additionally, they are designed as liquids and powders that can be reconstituted into liquids. Typically, liquid dose forms are designed for usage with elderly and pediatric patients. Excipients required for liquid dosage forms include a vehicle, stabilizer, and viscosity builder, as well as preservatives, sweeteners, colorants, and flavors. Additionally, solubilizers are needed for clear liquids, as well as suspending agents and emulsifying agents for suspensions and emulsions, respectively .Despite their many uses, liquid dosage forms are particularly preferred by the elderly and young children who have trouble swallowing pills or capsules. These also have scents that make them tasty and a more calming feeling as they travel down the throat.

ADVANTAGES OF LIQUID DOSAGE FORMS –

- Liquid dosage forms are most convenient to administer.
- People specially children having difficulty in swallowing solid dosage forms like tablets and capsules can easily swallow liquid.
- Our API [Active Pharmaceutical Ingredient] is more homogeneously dissolved in liquid dosage forms in comparison to solid.
- To get absorbed in the body drug must be in a solution form.
- The drug given to the patient in solution is more readily available for absorption and shows better efficacy in comparison to other dosage forms.
- Unlike tablets the dose in adjustable/flexible in syrup etc.
- They look more appealing to the eye because of attractive color and aesthetic appeal because of coloring agents.
- The bitter taste and odor is masked by sweetening and flavoring agents, hence they are more palatable.
- For few medication only liquid dosage form is preferred for ex antacids and cough relieving syrups.

DISADVANTAGES OF LIQUID DOSAGE FORMS-

- The physiochemical stability of liquid dosage forms is far less then that of solid dosage forms.
- So, they show more chemical degradation.
- They become very bulky so transporting them is a cumbersome process.
- Also storing them is required with special conditions of temperature and moisture.
- More preservatives are needed as they are more prone to microbial growth because of presence of syrup.
- The dose is administered accurately when the patient measures the appropriate volume, which increases the likelihood of variability.
- This can be a major problem for individuals who have eye problems, arthritis, or difficulty reading the numbers on their oral dosing syringe and medicine cup.
- Container breakage is a problem which not only wastes the dosage form but also a economic loss.
- **EXCIPIENTS USED IN LIQUID DOSAGE FORMS-**

First of all let we understand what is an excipient? Any substance or ingredient other then the active pharmaceutical ingredient which is required to formulate a dosage form is an excipient

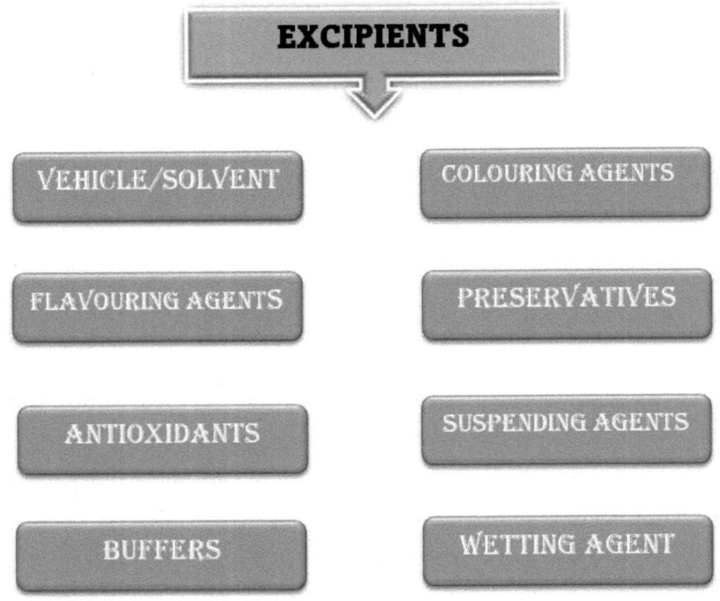

Excipients

SOLUBILITY ENHANCEMENT TECHNIQUES DOSAGE FORMS-

Excipients should be chosen carefully based on their physico-chemical properties, the characteristics of the active ingredient, and the mode of administration. Regulations, consistency of the substance, sources, pricing, availability, stability and compatibility difficulties, pharmacokinetic parameters, permeability traits, segmental absorption behavior, drug delivery platform, intellectual property issues, etc. all play a role in excipient selection. Understanding A excipients, their interactions, and process factors is essential for producing good pharmaceutical formulations. In order to create an oral liquid formulation that is stable, efficient, and appetizing, the choice of excipients is important. The final excipient choice for a given application is dependent on the results of compatibility testing, which give the manufacturer insight into potential interactions.

IDEAL PROPERTIES OF EXCIPIENTS-

1. Excipients function effectively for their intended application.
2. They should have no physiological activity.
3. They must be chemically and physically stable.
4. They ought to be less susceptible to machinery and procedures.
5. They should not be poisonous.
6. They must meet requirements for organoleptic qualities.
7.No impact on the drug's bioavailability.
8. The excipients must be devoid of harmful bacteria.
9. They must comply with the rules set forth by the regulating body.
10. They must be cost-effective.

FUNCTIONS OF EXCIPIENTS-

1. They could be included to keep the dose form's integrity.
2. They offer stability, support, or protection to the formulation.
3. They aid in creating sufficient formulation size for powerful drugs to help with precise dosing and handling.
4. They enhance the acceptability of the patient.
5. They help increase the drug's bioavailability.

6. They help to preserve and improve the formulation's overall safety and efficacy during its storage and use.

CLASSIFICATION-

The excipients are classified on the basis of their uses –

1.VEHICLE/SOLVENT –

- Liquid dosage forms may be prepared using aqueous solvents like ethyl alcohol, isopropyl alcohol, purified water, glycerin etc.
- The active pharmaceutical ingredient's (API) composition, physicochemical qualities, and the formulation's intended application all influence the choice of vehicle.
- Vehicles are important components used as a base in liquid pharmaceutical formulations in which medicines and other excipients are solvated or disseminated.
- They break the bonds which leads to decreased ionic charges, which raises the solute-solvent forces of attraction until they surpass solute-solute and solvent-solvent forces of attraction.

A.WATER- As impurities, water contains several dissolved and suspended particles. Inorganic impurities including sodium, potassium, calcium, magnesium, and iron salts in the form of chlorides, sulphates, and bicarbonates are among the dissolved impurities. Organic contaminants might be soluble or insoluble when present in purified water. The other pollutants in water are microorganisms. Less than 0.1% of the total solids are in drinkable water. This water ought to satiate IP specifications. Clear, odorless, colorless, and neutral drinking water that has a small pH variation from dissolved particles and gases is what IP considers appropriate.

B.ETHANOL- Next to water, ethanol—often referred to as "alcohol"—is the solvent most frequently employed in liquid medicinal formulations. It is typically employed as a hydro-alcoholic mixture to dissolve medications and excipients that are alcohol- and water-soluble. In numerous pharmaceutical processes and formulations, diluted ethanol, created by mixing equal amounts of Ethanol IP and Purified Water IP, is a very helpful solvent to dissolve poorly soluble compounds. Several production procedures in the pharmaceutical sector employ alcohol. Especially in alcohol gel for hands, it exhibits bactericidal activity and is frequently used as a topical disinfectant. Additionally, it is frequently utilised in liquid pharmaceutical preparations as a preservative and solvent.

C.GLYCEROL- Glycerol, which is also known as glycerin, is a clear, colourless liquid that has a thick, syrup-like consistency, is oily to the touch, is odourless, extremely sweet, and has a somewhat warm flavour. It progressively takes in moisture after being exposed to the air. The breakdown of vegetable, animal, or fixed oils yields glycerol, which contains at least 95% absolute glycerin. Insoluble in ether, chloroform, carbon disulfide, benzene, benzol, or fixed or volatile oils, it is soluble in water or alcohol in all amounts as well as a mixture of three parts alcohol and one part ether. Phosphoric Acid Elixir, Ferric Ammonium Acetate Solution, Tragacanth Mucilage, Boric acid Glycerin, Tannic acid Glycerin, and several extracts, syrups, and tinctures all use glycerin as a carrier.

2. COLOURING AGENTS-

Pharmaceutical products frequently contain (coloring agents) to standardize or enhance the color of the drugs already in use, to hide color changes and enhance appearance. Liquid coloring agents might have more sensitivity towards temperature change light and microbial contamination and powdered one have dusting issues and granules have solubility problems so the excipient should be carefully chosen keeping all these factors in mind. Examples-

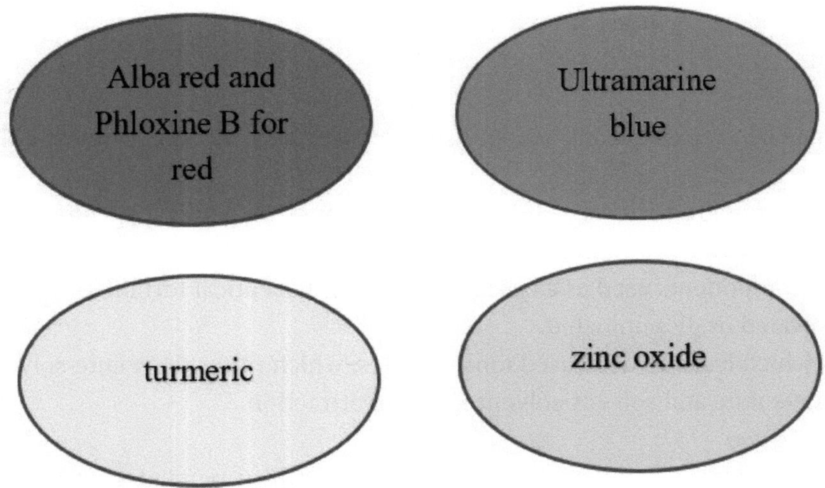

COLOURING AGENTS

3. FLAVOURING AGENT-

The flavoring agents are employed to mask the taste of the dosage form and make it more palatable

The flavor of a substance is an experience with numerous dimensions, including odor, subjective and objective judgements of taste and feeling factors like cooling sensation on.

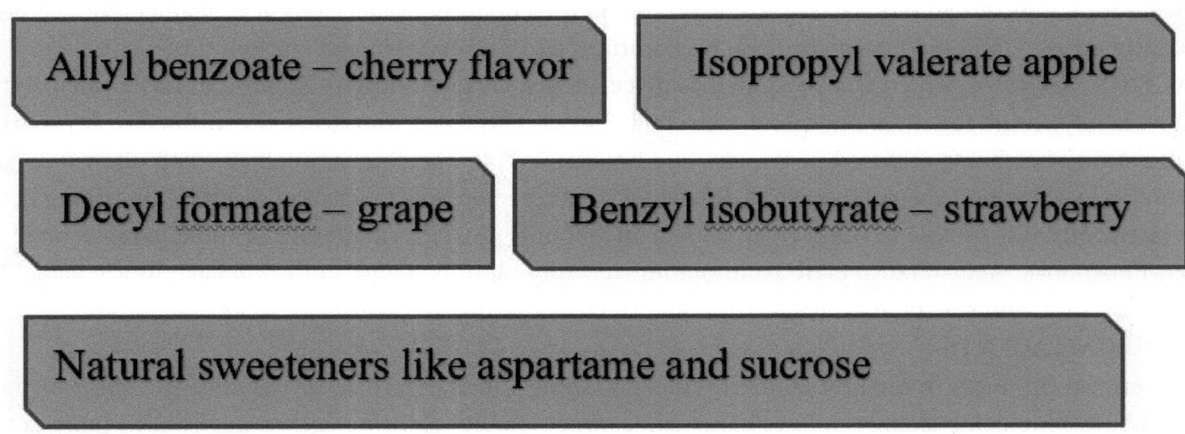

FLAVOURING AGENT

4. PRESERVATIVES-

Many liquid dosage forms like syrup contains all the vital components required for bacterial and fungal growth which not only diminishes the product quality but also toxic for human life. As we all know that liquid dosage forms being more prone to microbial contaminations so the must be added with preservative for preventing it from contamination and enhance its shelf life . As preservative inhibit the microbial growth.

The quantity of the preservative is can be decided according to the proportions of other ingredients. EXAMPLES-

NAME	CONCENTRATION [IN V/V]
• BENZOIC ACID	• 0.1% TO 0.2 %
• SODIUM BENZOATE	• 0.1% TO 0.2%
• ETHYL PARABEN	
• IMIDUREA METHYL PARABEN	• 0.001% TO 0.2% • 0.05% TO 0.18%

5. ANTIOXIDANTS –

Oxidation is basically defined as a process of addition of oxygen or loss of electron in a reaction. These reaction leads to release of free radicals or molecular oxygen which increases the risk of degradation.

So we antagonize this effect by using antioxidants which works by two mechanism the first one is by combining with the free radical to stop the chain reactions ex- butylated hydroxytoluene and second one is by using reducing agents like ascorbic acid.

6.Suspending agents-

In case liquid dosage forms the particles tend to form agglomerates that get heavy and settle down in the bottle and the amount of API that is to be given is significantly fluctuated so to avoid this problem we use suspending agents which diminishes the attraction between the particles by creating an energy barrier.

Ex – cellulose polymers like methyl cellulose, ethyl cellulose; clays like bentonite and gums like acacia, tragacanth etc.

7. BUFFERS/ pH STABILISERS-

An important consideration is the pH of liquid formulations, especially those intended for oral delivery. The pH assists in preserving the formulation by preventing unintended changes during storage. Therefore, buffers, which have the ability to stop pH changes, are included in the majority of formulations to manage possible pH alterations. In bases, hydrogen ions are given as opposed to being bound by buffers. Between 0.05 and 0.5 M of concentration is typically adequate, while between 0.01 and 0.1 M of buffer capacity is typically required. The selection of an appropriate buffer should take into account the stability of the medicine and excipients in the buffer, compatibility of the buffer with the container, and acceptability of the acid-base form for use in oral liquids.

As opposed to using separate buffers, a mixture of buffers has also been utilized to prepare a wide range of pH. It is significant to remember that not all buffers can be used with oral liquids. For instance, due to its toxicity, a boric acid buffer is not utilized in oral liquids. pH affects the formulation's stability when non-ionizable medicines are present. The buffer, however, can have a deleterious impact on the drug's and other excipients' solubility. The polarity of the salt and the solute together determine the outcome. Less polar organic salts can dissolve non-polar solutes, while polar salts can desolubilize them.

The possible interaction between excipients and drugs is controlled by the stabilizing effect of buffers. For instance, buffers containing sparingly soluble salts like carbonate, citrate, tartrate, and phosphate may precipitate with calcium ions. The pH of the solution determines this precipitation. Due to interactions with other elements of the solution, the activity of phosphate ions may be decreased. Temperature, ionic strength, dilution, and the presence of different co-solvents can all have an impact on the pH of a solution. For instance, it is well known that the pH of acetate buffers rises as the temperature rises, whereas the pH of boric acid buffers falls as the temperature rises. It is crucial to be aware that the medicine in solution may function as its own buffer.

Examples: Phosphate buffers, Acetate buffers, Citric acid Phosphate buffers etc.

8.WETTING AGENTS -

Any dosage form must first have a homogenous dispersion of solute particles in a liquid medium. Such pharmacological formulations frequently employ wetting agents. They are kept away from moving vehicles by the air adsorbing at solid particle surfaces. Even highly dense particles float on the surface of the car. To scatter them evenly in vehicles, the air at surfaces must be totally displaced. Wetting agents aid in the removal of adsorbed air, which in turn facilitates the liquid vehicle's entry into the pores and capillaries of the particles.

Hydrophilic-lipophilic balance (HLB) values for wetting agents range from 7 to 9. It is vital to know the minimum surface tension that can be achieved, regardless of the amount of agent used, when choosing a wetting agent for any liquid composition. Aside from that, it's also crucial to know how much surface tension is depressed at a certain agent concentration and how long it takes an agent to reach equilibrium.

Wetting agents utilized for the purpose shouldn't cause any unintended changes to the medications' or other excipients' potential action or efficacy.

SOLUBILITY- It is defined as the ability of the solute to get dissolved into a solution resulting in formation of a homogeneous solution. To be in a solution form is the basic criteria. The solubility of any entities is dependent upon various factors like temperature, pressure, PH etc.

SOLUBILITY ENHANCEMENT TECHNIQUES-

Few medicaments having very good therapeutic value are not having good solubility in the vehicles so their solubility needs to be enhanced.There are various techniques to enhance the solubility –

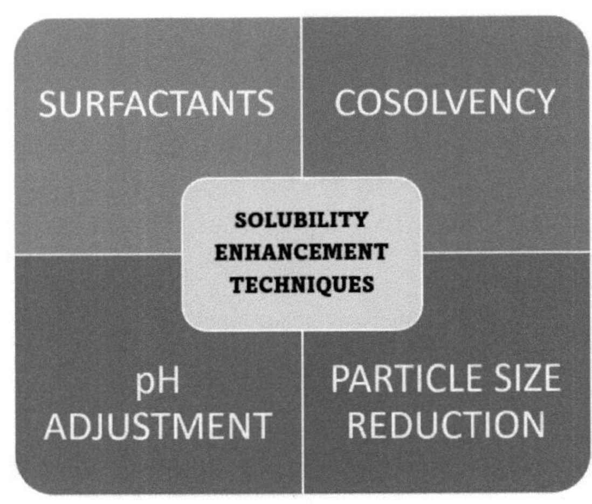

SOLUBILITY ENHANCEMENT TECHNIQUES

1.SURFACTANTS-

Sometimes the solubility problems arise due to the interfacial tension arising at surface of solute and solvents so surfactants are used to reduce this surface tension which leads to better wetting and solvation interaction.

Surfactants have a hydrophilic[polar] head and hydrophobic[non-polar] tail Benzalkonium chloride ,cetylpyridiniumchloride, polyoxymethylene esters includes polyethylene glycol[PEG40,PEG-50,PEG-55] and ethers of fatty alcohols are the examples of some commonly used surfactants.

2.COSOLVENCY –

- Cosolvents are water miscible solvents that can be added to a solution of a medicine that is weakly water soluble to boost the drug's solubility.
- Co-solvents are solutions with increased solubility for weakly soluble chemicals that are made up of water and one or more water miscible solvents.
- Ex- Propylene glycol, PEG 300, and ethanol
- Drugs with limited solubility can be delivered parenterally and orally using co-solvent formulations.
- Using a co-solvent is appropriate for poorly soluble chemicals that are lipophilic or highly crystalline and have a high solubility in the solvent mixture.

3. pH Adjustment

- Drugs that are poorly soluble in water but include molecular components that may be protonated (base) or deprotonated (acid) may be dissolved in water by changing the pH.
- In theory, both parenteral and oral administration can involve pH adjustment.
- Following oral administration, the degree of solubility is likely to be affected as the drug travels through the intestines since the pH of the stomach is between 1 and 2 and that of the duodenum is between 5 and 7.5.
- The most suitable ionizable chemicals are those that remain stable and soluble despite pH adjustment. The different chemical kinds include zwitter ions, bases and acids
- Both crystalline and lipophilic poorly soluble molecules can benefit from it.

4.PARTICLE SIZE REDUCTION-

- The size of the particle plays very important role when it comes to solubility.
- The surface area to volume ratio rises as a particle gets smaller.
- Greater contact with the solvent is made possible by the bigger surface area resulting into increasing solubility.
- Machines used for size reduction are ball mill, rotary cutter mill , roller mill, fluid energy mill, hammer mill etc.

CHAPTER VIII

MONOPHASIC LIQUID DOSAGE FORM

MONOPHASIC LIQUID DOSAGE FORMS

3.1 INTRODUCTION:

A monophasic liquid dosage form is essentially a liquid formulation that comprises several components in one phase system.

As a result of the homogeneous nature of the combination, it is regarded as true solution. The solute, which is present in a lesser quantity than the solvent, and the solvent, which is present in a larger quantity, are the two basic components of a solution.

Both internal and external applications of these solutions are possible. These all have a basis of either aqueous or non-aqueous solvents.

ADVANTAGES :

1. Due to the homogeneity of these dose forms, it is simple for the medication to be dispersed evenly throughout the body.
2. They are absorbed much more quickly than pills and capsules since they are in solution form.
3. Paediatric, geriatric, and psychiatric patients who have trouble ingesting solid dose forms like pills and capsules are especially in need of solutions.
4. Additionally, they may be coloured, sweetened, and flavoured.

DISADVANTAGES:

1. Compared to solid dosage forms, it is less stable since they deteriorate more quickly.
2. It might be difficult to disguise the unpleasant taste of some medications.

3.2 CLASSIFICATION:

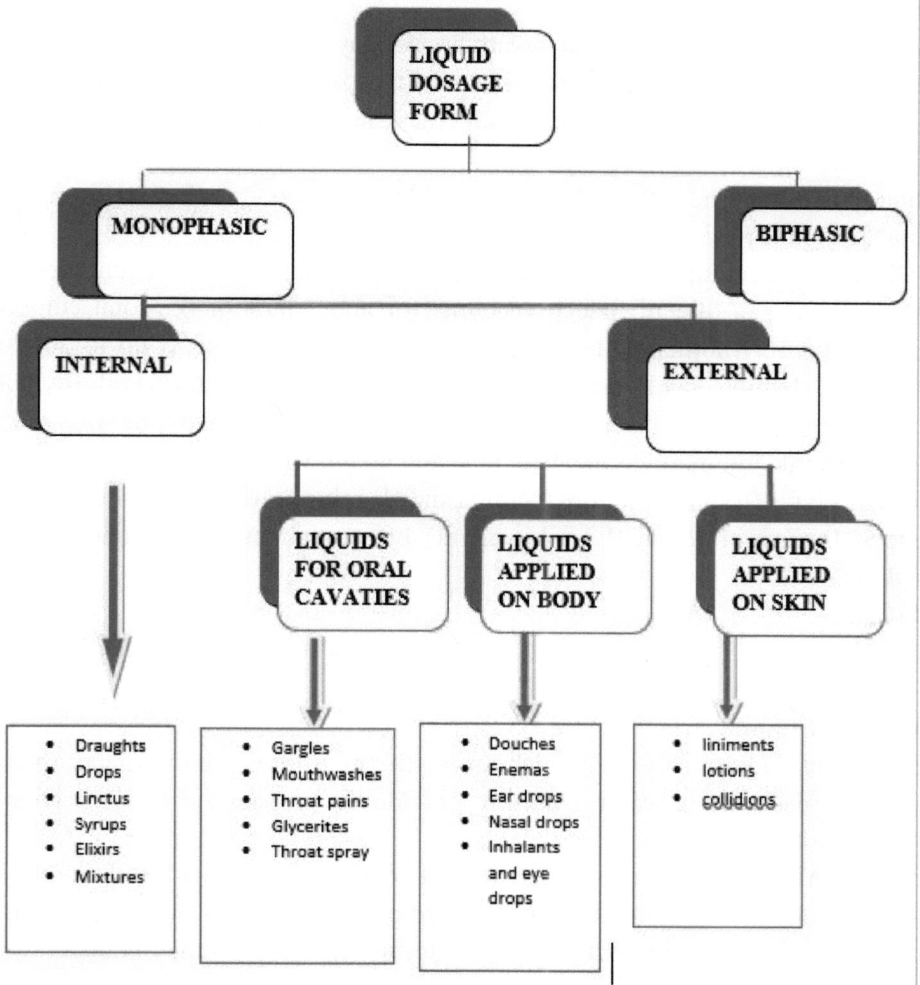

3.3 LIQUIDS FOR ORAL CAVITIES

3.3.1 GARGLES :

Gargles are clear aqueous solutions that are used to treat throat infections. These are diluted with warm water before use. They are used in a way to make the medication come into contact with the mucosal surface of the throat, where it is left for a short period of time before being spat out of the mouth.

Gargles may contain some therapeutic agents like antibiotics, antiseptics, analgesics, deodorants, and astringents.

Gargles have to be administered in transparent fluted glass bottles with plastic screw caps on them.

The label should provide instructions for diluting the gargle before use.

METHOD OF PREPARATION :

In a beaker, combine phenol glycerin and a tiny amount of amaranth solution. Add 3/4" of water and stir once more. Fill the measuring cylinder with the contents. Use water to wash and adjust to the desired volume. Place the label on the bottle, close it with a closure, and transfer to a clean bottle.

Gargles are often made by dissolving drug ingredients with the right excipients in a solvent, filtering, and adding the right excipients. Prepare Tablets or Granules as indicated in the case of solid preparations that must be dissolved prior to use. You can ingest herbal gargles to get a secondary systemic impact. Before using, many gargles need to be diluted with water.

Examples : phenol gargles, potassium chlorate and phenol gargles.

3.3.2 MOUTH WASHES :

Mouthwashes are aqueous solutions used to clean and deodorise the mouth.

Some of the therapeutic substances present include antibiotics or astringents, alcohol, glycerin, sweeteners, surfactants, flavouring, and colouring additives.

Mouthwashes are designed to eliminate bad breath in he ways. First, they relieve it by killing the bacteria responsible for producing the foul odo The best of these products prevent bad breath for as long as eight hours. The secon way that mouthwashes help reduce bad breath is by masking the odour. This is a less effective method which lasts no more than 30 minutes.

Example : alkaline phenol mouth wash, hydrogen peroxide mouth wash, buffer sodium perborate mouth wash, compound sod. Chloride mouth wash.

CONTENTS : Glycerol, sweetening, flavouring, soaps, colouring, and astringent are some of the active constituents . Deionized water, a diluent, which accounts for about 50% of the total composition, is often the mouthwash's main constituent. Another diluent commonly included in formulas up to 20% of which is alcohol. Ingredients like phenols, thymol, salol, tannic acid, hexachlorophene, chlorinated thymols, and quaternary ammonium compounds are used as antibacterial agents in mouthwash formulations. Common flavorings include eugenol, menthol, peppermint, and methyl salicylate. Blue and green, which are FDA-approved and verified, are the most frequently utilized colors. To add even more foaming and cleaning power, some mouthwash recipes also contain a synthetic detergent. Sodium chloride mouth wash contains different chemical components in it.

FORMULA AMOUNT

Sodium chloride 2gm

Sodium bicarbonate 1gm

Amaranth solution 2ml

Peppermint water up to 100ml

The mouthwash contains sodium chloride, which makes the mixture isotonic. Amaranth solution is utilised as a colouring ingredient and peppermint water is used to provide the preparation a nice flavour and odour. Sodium carbonate aids in the dissolution of mucus.

METHOD OF PREPARATION : In a beaker, combine 3/4 volume of water with sodium bicarbonate and sodium chloride to dissolve. Mix well before adding the concentrated peppermint emulsion chloroform water. Transfer the contents to the measuring cylinder, then use the leftover water to adjust the volume. Transfer the mixture to a bottle, then seal it and apply a label.

Mouth washes should be administered in clear, fluted bottles. The mouthwash bottle should be labelled with instructions for dilution before use.

Mouth washes should be stored in clear fluted bottles.

3.3.1THROAT PAINT :

During any mouth or throat infections, mucosal surfaces are coated with throat paints. These throat paints are basically viscous liquid preparations.

Antibiotics, iodides, phenol, and tannic acid are just a few of the medications that are included in these throat paints.

These throat paints are viscous because of the presence of commonly used base called glycerin.

They are thickened to add viscosity, which allows the medicine to stay in touch with the mucosal membrane long enough to exert its full effect.

The proper container for throat paints should have a broad aperture and an airtight seal. These bottles need to have stoppers as well.

They need to be kept in cool areas. The warning "not to be ingested in large amounts" should be written on the containers.

Example: compound iodine paint, crystal violet paint etc.

Uses: Applying iodine to the external throat can help with tonsillitis, pharyngitis, laryngitis, and other disorders. It can also lessen throat pain and perhaps prevent or even cure throat infections. When the solution is painted internally on throat tissue, it has been found that the effect of iodine paint in cases of throat infections is significantly larger. We must be careful to choose a suitable formulation when utilising this kind of preparation. Although most people consider iodine to be safe, some people should avoid it, and it should not be taken with particular drugs. Iodine should not be taken by anyone who has Hashimoto's autoimmunity thyroid disease or an overactive thyroid. Chronic toxicity may manifest when iodine intake exceeds 1.1 mg/day, according to the Merck manual. People who may have an iodine allergy should also take extra care. A quick test is to apply a very small amount to the inner thigh's skin and watch for small blisters to form within a few hours. If blisters do develop, you can be allergic to iodine paint or experience an adverse reaction to it. To kill bacteria, iodine throat paint is used. It can be used to soothe ulcers and sore throats.

Compound iodine paint is also called as Mandl's throat paint. It contains different chemical components in it, those are :

FORMULA AMOUNT

Potassium iodide 25gm

Iodine 12.5gm

Alcohol 90%v/v 40ml

Water 25ml

Peppermint oil 4ml

Glycerol up to 1000ml

Potassium iodide is used so that on combination with iodine it forms potassium triiodide which is soluble in water. Iodine present in it acts as an antiseptic, it even penetrates in the pores and show germicidal effect. Alcohol acts as a preservative, water is the solvent and peppermint oil acts as a flavouring agent.

METHOD OF PREPARATION ;

1. Iodine should be triturated in a glass mortar to obtain a fine powder so that it may be precisely weighed.
2. Potassium iodide should be dissolved with water. Add iodine powder to this mixture, and dissolve by stirring.
3. Mix half of the glycerin portion and the peppermint oil in the alcohol.
4. This solution should be added to the iodide and potassium iodide solution mentioned above while being continuously stirred. The final volume should then be adjusted using the leftover glycerin.

3.4 LIQUIDS APPLIED ON BODY

3.4.1 EARDROPS:

Ear drops are liquid solutions designed to be instilled into the ear with a dropper. The medications are dissolved or suspended in the liquid.

Propylene glycol, polyethylene glycol, and glycerin are the three most often used vehicles out of all those that are employed.

Since ear secretions are primarily fatty, water is not recommended as a medium due to mixing issues.

Ear drops are typically used to treat minor infections, dry weeping surfaces, soften wax, and clean out the ear.

Ear drops are delivered in appropriate plastic containers or in coloured fluted bottles with droppers. "For outdoor use only" labels must be placed on the containers.

Example: sodium bicarbonate ear drops, chloramphenicol ear drops, chloromycetin ear drops etc.

Sodium bicarbonate ear drops are basically used to relieve from itching.

Advantages:

1. They may not always be sterile
2 Used to remove earwax buildup or to treat infections.
3. They are less dangerous than systemic treatment
4. They bypass the systemic circulation and are administered directly to the affected organ.
5. Drugs administered using ear drops have few side effects, including local itchiness and allergies.
6. Typically, they are less expensive than comparable systemic drugs.

Disadvantages:

1. There is a small chance that the ear being treated has a perforated eardrum, which could result in irreversible hearing loss.
2. Long-term use carries a small risk of dizziness.

3. Effective administrative abilities are necessary.
4. The usage of an ear drop could cause pain.

3.4.2 NASAL DROPS:

Nasal drops are aqueous solutions that are instilled into the nostrils using a dropper. Because of their antibacterial, local analgesic, or vasoconstrictor characteristics, they are frequently utilised.

The vasoconstrictor medications currently available help to clear nasal congestion.

Earlier oily preparations using liquid paraffin or vegetable oils as the vehicle were employed to extend the effect of the medicine, but the use of oily vehicles in the formulation of nasal drops is now discouraged because on continuous usage, the oil slows the ciliary movement of the nasal mucosa or drops of oil may enter the trachea and cause lipoid pneumonia. So it's recommended that nasal drops be delivered by an aqueous vehicle.

Whenever possible, nasal drops should be made iso-osmotic with 0.9% sodium chloride; this means that the tonicity should be equivalent to normal saline, the pH range should be 5.5-7.5, with mild buffer capacity, and the viscosity should not be greater than that of nasal mucus; this is because nasal secretions are similar in viscosity to nasal mucus; this can be accomplished by adding a thickening agent, such as 0.5% methyl cellulose.

They should be administered in coloured fluted bottles with a dropper-attached screw top. These drops should be dispensed in small quantities that is 10 to 25 ml.

Example : betnisol N nasal drops, decon nasal drops, diconal nasal drops etc.

Advantages:

1. suitable for medications that readily penetrate mucosal membranes and enter the bloodstream.
2. By directly entering the bloodstream, gastrointestinal damage and hepatic first pass metabolism are avoided.
3. Drugs have a predictable bioavailability and are quickly absorbed.
4. Drug plasma concentrations and absorption rates are equivalent to intravenous delivery.
5. They are simple, practical, and secure to use.
6. They might quickly reach therapeutic medication concentrations in the brain and spinal cord (CNS).
7. Injections are more expensive than these.

Disadvantages:

1. a small number of drugs that can be administered by nasal drops.
2. Numerous drugs lack the necessary concentration to produce appropriate dosage quantities.
3. Absorption is impacted by mucosal health.
4. The sinus membranes may be permanently harmed by repeated use.
5. The majority of nasal drops have a number of adverse reactions, including weariness, nosebleeds, throat irritation, and cough.

3.4.3ENEMAS:

Enemas can be aqueous or oily solutions or suspensions and are administered in the colon or rectum for cleansing, medicinal, or diagnostic purposes

They are used for their sedative, anthelminthic, anti-inflammatory, purgative, or nutritional properties.

These enemas are used for various purposes. For example:

- **Cleansing enemas** are used to evacuate feaces in constipation or before an operation. These function in two ways: first, by promoting peristalsis, and other is by lubricating impacted faeces. Peristalsis can be promoted by various drugs. For Large volume: Plain water Soft soap Turpentine enemas whereas for Small volume (Osmotic retention) Sodium phosphate enema, Magnesium sulphate enema, Sorbitol Sodium chloride are used. Lubrication of the impacted faeces is done by Olive oil enemas, Araches oil Enemas, and Glycerin enemas.
- **Therapeutic enemas** are used for therapeutic purposes such as sedation, anthelminthics, and anti-inflammatory. Medications including chloral hydrate paraldehyde, quassia, and corticosteroids are contained in them.
- **Diagnostic enemas** are utilized for diagnostic purposes, such as for lower bowel X-ray examination. For instance, barium sulphate enemas.

- Enemas available in disposable plastic bags are said to be **disposable enemas**. They consist of retention enemas containing prednisolone as well as evacuant enemas using magnesium sulphate.

Typically, solutions are administered as an enema in volumes ranging from 500 ml to 1000 ml, depending on the patient's age and health. The commercially available concentrated enemas, however, are administered in modest doses of 100 to 200 ml. Enemas with a large volume should be warmed to body temperature before use.

TYPES OF ENEMAS

1. **Evacuant enemas**
2. **Retention enemas**

Evacuant enemas : these can be given up to 2L. A normal evacuation enema consists of 500 ml of water and 25 g of soft soap. It is supplied in plainscrew-capped bottle. For insoluble particles in enemas, starch mucilage can be utilised as an emollient and suspending agent. Similar uses for sodium carboxymethylcellulose are possible.

Retention enemas : Retention enemas usually have volumes under 100 ml. In general, rectal injections are used as a base anaesthetic prior to surgery.

For instance Thiopentone sodium, is administered at a dose of 40 mg per kg of body weight and is dissolved in 30 ml of sterile water. It must be made freshly. Sometimes, a 10% solution of paraldehyde in sodium chloride solution is administered rectally.

Preauction : large volume enemas should be warmed to body temperature before administration.

Example : laxicon enema

Practo-clyss enema

USES :

Enemas are rectal injections used to induce vomiting, absorb nutrients into the body, treat localised illness sites, and perform diagnostic procedures.

The GIT is visualised. Enemas are used to administer nutritional, sedative, anthelmintic, anti-inflammatory, purgative, stimulant, or nourishing drugs to the colon.

3.5 INTERNAL DOSAGE

3.5.1 SYRUPS :

Syrups are concentrated aqueous sucrose solutions that are sweet and viscous. Other medications and chemicals are also present in this solution.

Normally, sucrose is used to make syrup, however dextrose or polyols, such as glycerin, sorbitol, or other polyhydric alcohols, are often substituted to prevent the crystallisation of sucrose or to increase the solubility of medications and other additions.

1. Medicated syrup

Essentially, syrup or simple syrup is the preparation name for the sucrose solution made solely with purified water. Thus depending on the substance added to this syrup its of two types :

2. Flavouring syrup

Medicated syrup : Medicated syrup is the name given to a preparation when it includes a medicated ingredient in the syrup.

Flavouring syrup : Flavouring syrups are those that does not include any medicine but do contain a variety of fragrant or pleasantly flavoured ingredients in the syrup. They are employed to cover up the unpleasant flavour of bitter medications.

In order to prevent contamination during preparation, clean containers must be used along with this sucrose and purified water that is devoid of foreign chemicals should be selected . While mould, yeast, and other microbes can develop in sucrose solutions that are too diluted, their growth is typically inhibited when the concentration of sucrose is 65% weight by weight or higher. However, a saturated solution can cause sucrose to crystallise.

If significant quantities of syrup are to be created, they must be properly maintained to prevent contamination. Only limited quantities of syrup that may be consumed within a few months should be prepared. Syrups can be kept fresh for a long time at temperatures under 25°C. Preservatives such glycerin, methyl paraben, benzoic acid, and sodium benzoate can be added to diluted solutions.

Artificial syrups made from artificial sweeteners are being offered in the market. Since they don't contain any carbohydrates, they can be given to diabetic patients more easily than syrups made from sugar. Additionally, they are less stable than syrups made with sugar.

Syrups are employed in the formulation of antibiotics, antitussives, antihistamines, vitamins, and analgesic/antipyretics.

Examples : Benadryl syrup

Corex cough syrup

Crocin syrup

Advantages :

1. Syrups can be conveniently administered and have the capacity to mask a drug's unpleasant taste.
children.
2. The thick consistency of the syrup provides a calming effect on the throat's inflamed tissues.
3. contain very little alcohol, if any.
4. Simple to change the dosage based on a child's weight
5. able to withstand microbial growth
6. appealing to young people.

Disadvantages :

1. Patients who need to eat less caloric food should be mindful of
sugar content in the syrup.
2. Patients who routinely consume syrups are at risk for dental caries.
3. Patients with diabetes should not use.
4. If the bottle of sugar is left open, crystallisation occurs.

3.5.2 ELIXIR :

Elixirs are clear, pleasant, sweetened hydroalcoholic liquid preparations intended for oral administration. It is typically less sweet and viscous than syrup.

The main ingredient of syrup are :

- Water
- Ethanol
- Glycerin
- Sorbitol
- Propylene glycol
- Colouring agents : amaranth, compound tartrazine
- Flavouring agents : lemon spirit, compound orange spirit
- Sweetening agents: invert sugar, sodium saccharin
- Preservative : 20% alcohol as vehicle

TYPES OF ELIXIR

1. **Medicated elixir**: The medicated elixirs typically include highly potent medications like antibiotics, antihistamines, and sedatives.
2. **Non medicated elixir** : By using flavouring and sweetening agents, the bitter and nauseating taste of some medications can be covered up. The unmedicated elixirs are utilised for flavouring and are used as vehicles

Example : Formulation of phenobarbital elixir

FORMULA

phenobarbital 4g

orange oil 0.25ml

propylene glycol 100ml

Alcohol 200ml

sorbitol solution 600ml

colour qs

purified water 1000ml

Some other **examples of marketed elixir** are : betonin (vitamin B complex) elixir, cadiphylate elixir, ephedrine compound elixir.

Elixirs should be stored in firmly closed, light-resistant containers in a cool area because they typically contain volatile oils and alcohol, both of which degrade in the presence of air and light.

Advantages :

1. Keep the components that are soluble in alcohol and water in solution.
2. They are stable.
3. Simple solution procedure makes it simple to prepare.
4. Compared to syrups, elixirs have low viscosity.
5. Due to the low concentration of sucrose, which causes viscosity, they flow more easily.

Disadvantages :

1. less successful than syrups at hiding the taste of medications.
2. contains alcohol and emphasises the salty flavour of bromides.

Components :

Elixir's principal ingredients, along with those of the medicine, are water and alcohol. Aside from that to improve medicine solubility, product stability, palatability, and patient compliance, additional ingredients such glycerine, sorbitol, propylene glycol, preservatives, and flavouring compounds are also used. The solvents are frequently employed to make the medicinal ingredient more soluble as well as to

cover up an unpleasant taste in the dose form. Glycerine is used to increase a drug's solubility or sweeten a preparation, such as phenobarbital elixir USP.

Method of preparation :

Elixirs are easier to make than syrups due to the fact that they contain

fewer components that need to dissolve in larger quantities. if the mixture contains water and

The following process is typically used with components that are alcohol soluble.

1. Dissolve all of the water-soluble components in the water.
2. Add sucrose to the aforementioned solution and let it dissolve fully.
3. Put all the ingredients in alcohol that will dissolve in alcohol.
4. The first solution should be added to the second.
5. Elixir can be made transparent by filtering it and adding water to the final volume.

3.6 LIQUIDS APPLIED ON SKIN

3.6.1 LINIMENTS:

Liniments are preparations that are liquid or semi-liquid and intended to be applied topically to the skin. They could be alcoholic, oily, or an emulsion.

Two different types of solvents are utilised in the case of monophasic (solution) liniments:

1. **Alcohol** - Soap liniment
   - Aconite liniments.
2. **Oil**- Camphor Liniments
   - Methyl Liniments

Liniments containing substances have following properties:

- Analgesic
- Rubefacient
- Counter Irritants
- Soothing
- Stimulating

Liniments are often applied to the skin through friction and rubbing. They must not be applied to skin that has been damaged that is the broken skin.

Liniments acts as an irritant, counter-irritant and rubefacient.

Agents or compounds known as irritants create inflammation in the area to which they are applied rather than immediately destroying tissues. Rubefacients are chemicals that cause swelling and redness in the area where they are applied, causing the earliest signs of irritation.Counter-irritants are substances that are administered locally to irritate healthy skin in an effort to lessen or relieve another irritation or chronic pain. They appear to function by causing an inflammatory reaction, which increases blood flow to the injured location.

Containers should bear a label, " for external use only."

They should be stored in tightly closed containers.

Example : turpentine liniment, methyl salicylate liniment etc.

Patients with arthralgia (joint pain), myalgia (muscle pain), fibrositis (ligamental pain), and sprains are treated topically with turpentine liniment.

3.6.2LOTIONS :

Usually designed for external application to the skin, lotions are suspensions, dispersions, aqueous or alcoholic solutions. They are applied directly to the skin without rubbing using any absorbent material, such as cotton wool, or cotton wool or gauze that has been soaked in lotion.

When shake lotion is applied to the skin, the water evaporates, leaving a medication residue. The impact of evaporation is cooling. On the inflamed area, lotions are administered.

Alcohol is used to improve cooling and expedite (fasten) drying. The addition of glycerin helps keep skin moist for sufficient time. To aid in dispersion, a suspending agent may be utilized.

If no preservative is used during preparation, certain lotions can develop mould and bacteria. Care must be taken to prevent contamination during lotion manufacture, even if a preservative is added.

In colored fluted bottles, lotions ought to be administered. The container has to say "For external usage only" on it.

Examples : calamine lotion, oily calamine lotion, salicylic acid lotion and zinc sulphate lotion.

Lotions Containing Insoluble Substances

When a lotion comprises insoluble or non-diffusible ingredients, it must be dispensed in lotions similar to mixtures , which means adding three suspending agents. Tragacanth and other sticky gummy suspending agents are inappropriate for this use.

Therefore As suspending agents, bentonite and aluminium hydroxide gel are occasionally utilised.

The best illustration of a lotion containing an insoluble ingredient is calamine lotion. Calamine, zinc oxide, bentonite, sodium citrate, liquid phenol, glycerin, and purified water are all ingredients in this lotion.

Calamine is an non-diffusible and insoluble chemical. It has astringent, calming, and protecting properties.

Uses : This cream serves as an astringent and a sunburn preventative. It acts as a soother and provides comfort from discomfort and itching during skin irritation. Additionally, it treats eczema and ringworm infections.

Typically, lotions are liquid suspensions or dispersions meant to be applied topically to the skin. They could be prepared using the techniques below.

1. Trituration: Using high-speed mixers or homogenizers to thoroughly blend the ingredients into a paste before adding the remaining liquid phase slowly or in increasing amounts. One well-known example is calamine lotion, which is made up of finely powdered insoluble particles that are kept in more or less permanent suspension by the presence of suspending agents and/or surface active agents.

2. Chemical reaction: By altering the liquid's chemical composition, lotions can be made.
White Lotion, for instance, is a recently created composition that doesn't have a
agent that suspends. O/W type formulations stabilised by an is the second formulation type.
Benzyl Benzoate Lotion is an illustration of a surface active agent.

3. Solution method : Some lotions are transparent liquids, and their active constituents are
Things that are water soluble. Consider the lotion containing dimethisoqun hydrochloride.
Most common example of lotion is calamine lotion. The use of each ingredient present in this lotion is :

1. **Calamine** : Basic zinc carbonate is combined with a sufficient amount of ferric oxide to create calamine, which gives pink colour. Dermatologists frequently recommend it to give lotions or creams a flesh-like colour.
2. **Zinc oxide** : Mild astringent, protecting, and antiseptic effects are provided by zinc oxide. Is frequently used in lotions, ointments, and dusting powders for the treatment of skin conditions and infections such eczema, ringworm, and psoriasis.
3. **Bentonite** : A naturally occurring, hydrated aluminium silicate is called bentonite. It is insoluble in water but expands to almost seven times its original size to generate a desired viscosity magma. In order to disperse insoluble compounds like calamine, it is therefore utilised as a suspending agent.
4. **Sodium citrate** : In order to keep the lotion from becoming very thick that is viscous sodium citrate is added. It functions as a buffer and keeps the pH at a level suitable for skin preparations.
5. **Liquid phenol** : Liquid phenol has antibacterial and local anaesthetic qualities that make it an effective antipruritic.
6. **Glycerin** : As a hygroscopic substance, glycerin maintains the moisture content of the skin and has a calming impact on it.

Example : caladryl lotion, Calderm lotion, Calamine lotion

QUESTIONS :

1. Define monophasic liquid dosage form.
2. What is the classification of monophasic liquid dosage form
3. Define gargles, mouthwashes and also give its formulation.
4. Illustrate one example of throat paint and mention the uses of each component added to it.
5. Explain various techniques by which lotions can be prepared.

CHAPTER IX

Suspension

Suspension

Suspensions are heterogeneous systems in which solids are dispersed in liquids. Suspensions are the biphasic liquid dosage form in which finely divided solid particles are ranging from 0.5 to 5.0 microns are suspended in a liquids or semi-solid dosage form. There are two phases, one is the dispersion phase and the second is the dispersion medium or continuous phase and discontinuous phase. The solid particles are present in the discontinuous phase whereas the liquids are present in the continuous phase. They are unstable in nature. It may/may not exhibit the Tyndall effect. In this, we can see the solid particles from our naked eyes.

In suspension, particles will get settle down after some time, and shake to redispersion the solid particles again. It can be separated by filtration.

Examples of suspension

- Milk of magnesia
- Muddy water
- Flour in water
- Sand particles suspended in water
- Chalk suspended in water

Ideal features of suspension dosage form:

- The product of the suspension should be chemically, physically and microbiologically stable.
- Pharmaceutical suspensions should be aesthetically pleasing in nature and should also have a pleasing odour, and a pleasing taste.
- Suspended particles should be small and uniform in size in order to give smooth, elegant products without any gritty texture.
- Suspensions must not be too viscous then it will be difficult to pour and to flow from a needle syringe.
- All the doses dispensed from given multi-dose containers should have acceptable constancy of drug content.
- Suspended particles should settle down slowly and the sediments produced on storage, if any, should readily redispersion upon gentle agitation of the container.
- Parenteral and ophthalmic suspensions should be sterilizing
- Parenteral suspensions should be isotonic and non-irritating

Advantages of suspension

- Used in drugs or medications
- They are used in paints
- Higher concentrations of drug
- It can improve the taste and odour of the drug.

Disadvantages of suspension

- Sedimentation of particles
- Making of dosage from will be tough
- The accurateness of the dose is impossible

- Bulky in nature

Classifications of suspension

1. **Classifications of suspensions depending on their route of administrations:**

- Oral suspensions: These are the suspensions which is given by the oral route.

  Examples: Paracetamol suspensions, Aluminium Hydroxide, and Magnesium Hydroxide Suspensions.

- Parenteral suspensions: These are the suspension which is given by the intramuscular and intravenous routes.

  Example: Sodium benzylpenicillin suspensions.

- Ophthalmic suspensions: These types of suspensions are used for eyes. The particle size should be very small, non-irritant in nature, sterile, and isotonic.
- Topical suspensions: These suspensions are used for the topical uses

  Example: Calamine lotions.

2. **Based on Proportion of Solid Particle:**

- Dilute suspension: It has 2 to10% solid in weight per volume(w/v).

  Example: Prednisolone acetate, Cortisone acetate, etc.

- Concentrated suspension: It has 50% solid in weight per volume(w/v).

  Example: Zinc oxide suspensions.

3. **Based on Size of Dispersed Particle:**

- Molecular Dispersions: This type of suspension particles in which size is less than 1 nm.
- Colloidal Dispersions: This type of suspension particles in which size is between 0.1-0.2 µm.
- Coarse Dispersions: This type of suspension particles in which size is greater than 0.2 µm.

Formulation of Suspensions

1. **Wetting agents:** These are added up to disperse solids in a continuous liquid phase. Example: Polysorbate 80, 20, etc.
2. **Suspending agent:** These are added up to floccule the drug particles.
3. **Thickeners:** These are added up to enhance the viscosity of the suspension.
   Example: gaur gum, xanthan gum.
4. **Buffers and pH adjusting agents:** These are added up to stabilize the suspensions to the desired pH range.
5. **Coloring agents:** These are added up to transmit the desired color to suspensions and to improve elegance.
6. **Preservatives:** These are added up to stop the microbial growth.

Components of Suspension Formulation

The pharmaceutical suspension must be physically and chemically stable over the required time, be easily get rediapers after shaking and easy to manufacture and be acceptable in use to the patient. Thus, in order to deal in-depth, with these requirements selection of suitable excipients is of prime importance in preparing good quality suspension.

The main components of any suspension are insoluble solid drug particles and liquid medium. The other includes excipients such as suspending agent, surfactant, sweetener, colors, buffers, antioxidants etc.

PREPARATION OF SUSPENSION

Different steps follow during the preparation of suspension are:

1. Grinding of insoluble material with a vehicle containing the wetting agent to get a smooth paste
2. Dissolve soluble ingredients in some portion of the vehicle and added into above step to obtain the slurry
3. Remove the slurry to the graduated cylinder
4. Wash out the mortar with some part of the vehicle
5. Add suspending agent or flocculating agent if any by mixing it into the vehicle
6. Finally, adjust the volume by vehicle

By this, we have formulated suspension.

Flocculated Suspensions

A flocculated suspension are the suspensions in which particles of the suspensions have processed flocculation. Flocculations are the process in which colloid in a suspension can be achieved by an aggregated form. Therefore, a flocculated suspension is collected of large aggregates and this type of suspension will lead to a rapid rate of sedimentation because of the large flocs.

Flocculated suspensions are the suspensions in which particle of dispersed phase comes together to form a bunch structure called floccules.

A flocculated suspensions are the suspension in which particles of the suspension have undergone flocculations. A flocculated suspension is collected of large aggregate and this type of suspension will show rapid rate of sedimentation.

Sedimentations are the settling down of accumulation of suspension to the bottom of the liquid.

Deflocculated Suspensions

A deflocculated suspensions are the suspensions in which no flocculations have taken place. Hence, there are no floccules in the suspension. When sedimentation occur, these single particles settle down in a deflocculated suspensions, dispersed particles exist as single units. The rate of sedimentation is slow since smaller particles will settle down slowly compare to the larger flocs. The final sediments have a smaller volume than a flocculated suspensions. The formation of the sediments in the bottom is known as caking.**Flo**

Method of preparations of flocculated and deflocculated suspensions are;

Direct incorporation/ dispersion method

1. In the proper volume of diluents (vehicle), dissolve the soluble component.
2. By blending, the solid therapeutic agent is distributed into the vehicle, before being corrected for volume.

Formulating a vehicle that is as wet and distributed as possible will facilitate easy wetting and is distributed in the solid phase. This can be attained by using both wetting agents and suspending agents.

Stability of Suspensions

Factors that will contribute to the stability of a suspensions include:

1. Small Particles Size:

- The reduced size of the dispersed particles will enhance the surface area of the solid.
- The higher the degree of subdivision of a given solid the larger would be the surface area.
- The increase in surface area also means an increase in the interface between the solids and liquids leading to an increase in the viscosity of a system.

2. Increasing the Viscosity:

The increased viscosity of the continuous phase can lead to the stability.

• The rate of sedimentations can be reduced by the increase in viscosity. Viscosity increases by the addition of thickening agents to the external phase.

• It is essential to note that the rate of release of a drug from a suspension is dependent on viscosity.

3.Temperature:

- Factor that negatively affects the stability and usefulness of pharmaceutical suspensions is the change in the temperature. Temperature change can lead to caking of the material

Methods for stabilizing suspension

Physical Stability are attained by keeping the particle in Brownian motion

a. Provide electric charge on surface of dispersed particles: The like charge on the particles will stop this joining together and thus it will be keeping a Brownian motion.
b. Maintain solvent sheath around the particle:

The solvent layer stop the particles joining and also to maintain Brownian motion.

Evaluation of Suspensions:

1. Sedimentation method
2. Rheological method
3. Electro kinetic method
4. Micromeritic system

Forms of suspensions

The common pharmaceuticalsuspension preparations are differentiated into suspensions, gels, magmas and milks, lotions, enemas, inhalations, and mixtures for oral use.

1. **Suspensions:** Simple suspensions are the insoluble solid dispersed in a liquid. The stability considerations suggest that the manufacture of drugs in dry form is ideal. They are reconstituted as suspensions using a suitable vehicle before administration, for example, Cephalexin Powder (Keflex) and Azithromycin
2. **Gels:** Gels are the semisolid two-phase systems containing of little inorganic particles suspended in a liquid medium to form a network of little discrete particles, for example, Aluminum Hydroxide Gel USP
3. **Magmas and Milks**: Magmas and milk are the aqueous suspensions of huge insoluble, inorganic drugs. Freshly prepared magmas and milks are thick and viscous and thus require no suspending agents, for example, Bentonite magma, Milk of Magnesia etc.
4. **Enemas**: Enema suspensions are fluid preparations containing un-dissolved solids in aqueous medium injected into the lower bowel by way of the rectum for retention or evacuation, for example, Mesalamine Rectal Suspension USP
5. **Inhalations:** Inhalation suspensions are fluid preparations containing sterile undissolved solids in suitable non-aqueous propellant or propellant mixture inhaled via jet nebulizer, for example, Budesonide Suspension
6. **Mixtures:** Mixtures are oral liquids containing one or more active pharmaceutical ingredients dissolved or dispersed in a suitable vehicle. Suspended solids may disport slowly on standing, but they are easily re-dispersed on agitation.
7. **Injections:** Suspension for injection contain less than 5% of sterile drug in solid form with mean diameter within 5-10 um dispersed in suitable liquid.

Pharmaceutical application of suspensions

- Drugs which have very less solubility are usually formulated as suspensions.
- Suspended dosage forms of insoluble medicaments are not difficult to swallow
- Insoluble derivatives in the suspensions are more palatable than soluble derivatives in the solution
- They behave as adsorbent of toxins in GIT in the form of powder

Example. Chalk and Kaolin

Evaluation of suspension

The following tests are carried out on suspension formulation to assure final quality of suspension:

1. **Appearance, color, odor and taste**
2. **Particle size**
3. **Microscopic photography for crystal growth.**
4. **Sedimentation rate**
5. **Sedimentation volume**
6. **Zeta potential**
7. **Ph**
8. **Stress test**
9. **Rheological measurement**
10. **Centrifugation Test**

Model Questions

1. What is suspension? Give classification of suspension
2. Write a note on:

a. Stability of suspension
b. Flocculated and deflocculated suspension

3. Write the advantages of suspension?
4. Write the disadvantage of suspension?
5. What are the various types of disperse system?
6. Give methods of preparation of suspension
7. What are the various stability problems of suspensions?
8. List the evaluation test on suspension

CHAPTER X

EMULSIONS

An emulsion is a colloidal mixture of two or more liquids that are immiscible in nature. In an emulsion, one liquid is diluted into the other. It is a biphasic system of two immiscible liquids where one liquid is dispersed as a small globule in the other. There are disperse phase and disperse medium. The dispersed liquids are also known as the Internal or Discontinuous phase, whereas the dispersion mediums are known as the external or continuous phase.

Emulsions are thermodynamically unstable mixture of two unmixable liquids. Emulsions are also called heterogenous systems or biphasic systems.

The particle size of the globules ranges from 0.1 to 10 microns. The globules remain dispersed for very short time and after that, there will be separation globules as soon it stands, because of this we add emulsifying agents so to make the globules scattered in the dispersion medium, therefore a stable product is formed.

Emulsions are used extremely in the medical field. They are used externally and internally.

Dermatological preparations like lotion and creams are formulated as emulsions.

Examples of emulsions –

- Milk, cream in this the dispersed phase is liquid and dispersed medium are liquid.

In emulsion both the disperse phase and medium are liquid.

<u>Classification of Emulsion</u>

Emulsion can be classified into four types:

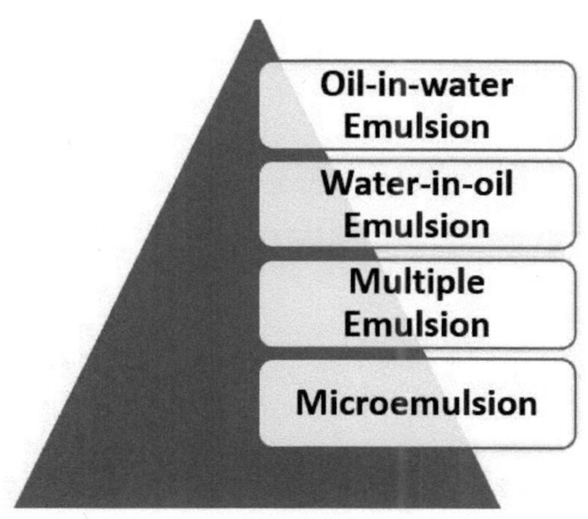

Classification of Emulsion

1. **Oil-in-water[o/w]**

In oil and water emulsions the oil is in the dispersed phase and water is in the dispersion medium. These are also known as aqueous emulsion.

The o/w type emulsion are non-greasy nature and can be easily removed from the body because of that it is used to formulate lotion, liniments and cream.

1. **Water-in-oil Emulsion**

Water and oil emulsions the water is in the dispersed phase and oil is in the dispersion medium. These are also known as oil emulsions.

W/O emulsion is greasy in nature, so it will be best to formulate the cold creams, moistures.

It has an ability to leave the skin oily do it will be best for dry skin problems.

3. **Multiple Emulsions**

Multiple emulsions are polydisperse system where both the oil in water and water in oil emulsion exists in the system simultaneously mannered.

They are also called "emulsion-within-emulsion" or "double emulsion". It will be either 'oil-in-water-in-oil' [o/w/o] type or 'water-in-oil-water' [w/o/w] type.

In oil-in-water-in-oil the o/w emulsion is dispersed in another oil phase. In o/w/o system an aqueous phase separate internal and oil phase separate external. O/W/O is a system in which water globules are surrounded in oil phase.

In water-in-oil-in-water the w/o emulsion is dispersed in another water phase. In w/o/w systems an organic phase separates internal and aqueous phase separate external. In this oil globules are surrounded by water phase.

It enhances bioavailability of drug.

4. **Microemulsion**

This system appears homogenous to naked eye. In microemulsion in which particle size of dispersed phase is less than 1μ. One phase system provides it thermodynamically stable.

It is less viscous compare to simple emulsion.

Emulsifying Agent

Emulsifying agents are also called emulgents of emulsifiers. Emulsifying agents reduce the interfacial tension between two phases which is oil and aqueous phase thus it makes them miscible with each other and form stable emulsion.

For making the stable emulsion it is tough to select a proper emulsifying agent. Sometimes we add more than one emulsifying agent instead of one because it's not necessary to have all the properties required for stable emulsion in one emulsifying agent.

Ideal properties of emulsifying agents

(1) Pharmaceutically acceptable emulsifiers must also be stable.

(i) It should be compatible with other constituents.

(ii) It should be non-poisonous.

(iv) It should have little or no odor, taste, or color.

(v) It should not interfere with the efficacy and stability of the active agent.

Classification of Emulsifying agents

1. Natural emulsifying agents:

- **Vegetable sources-** Tragacanthin, acacia, agar etc.
- **Animal sources-** Gelatin, Wool fat etc.

2. Semi-synthetic emulsifying agents: Methylcellulose, etc.

3. Synthetic emulsifying agents:

Anionic emulsifying agent: Sodium lauryl sulphate.

Cationic emulsifying agent: Benzalkonium Chloride.

- **Non-ionic emulsifying agent:** Sorbitan esters

- **Inorganic emulsifying agent:** Bentonite, magnesium oxide

<u>**Tests for identification of type of emulsion**</u>

Five tests for the identification of type of emulsion:

1. Dilution Test
2. Conductivity Test
3. Dye-Solubility Test
4. Cobalt Chloride Test
5. Fluorescence Test

1. **Dilution Test**

Take a test tube and add few drops of emulsion and dilute it with drops of oil. If the emulsion is diluted in the oil, then it is w/o type but if oil get separate out then it is o/w type of emulsion. Similarly, if the emulsion is diluted in water, then it is o/w type emulsion.

2. **Conductivity Test**

In this test we know that water is an excellent conductor of electricity and oil is non-conductor of electricity. So, the test is performed by immersing a pair of electrodes which is attached to an electric bulb into an emulsion. If it is o/w type emulsion then the bulb will glow because water is an excellent conductor of electricity

3. **Dye-Solubility Test**

Tests are conducted by mixing an emulsion with a water-soluble dye like amaranth and observe the results through a microscope. If it appears red continuous phase then it is a o/w type of emulsion. A Sudan III or Scarlet red C is added to an oil emulsion it causes a red continuous phase, which shows that the oil is not emulsified.

4. **Cobalt Chloride Test**

A filter paper is immersed in cobalt chloride solution and then immersed in an emulsion and dried it color changes from blue to pink then it is a o/w type emulsion.

5. **Fluorescence Test**

When an emulsion exhibits spotty fluorescence when it is exposed to ultra violet rays then it shows a o/w type emulsion and when it shows continuous fluorescence then it shows w/o type emulsion.

Methods of Preparation

The formulation of emulsion depends on the scale at which it is formulated.

On a small scale, mortar and pestle can be used although their efficiency is lowered. To get control of this disadvantage small electric mixers are used but care must be provided to stay away from excessive entrapping of air.

For large-scale productions mechanical stirrers are used to allowed a managed agitation and shearing stress to make safe emulsions.

The common methods by which we can formulate emulsion is by:

1. Trituration method

2. Bottle method

1. Trituration method:

It contains dry gum method and wet gum method

? Dry Gum Method

This method is also known as the 4:2:1 method because these ratios shows the proportions of oil: water: gum acacia needed for the preparation of primary emulsion.

1. Triturate the acacia powder and the oil into a moist-free mortar.
2. Measure the water for the primary emulsion and straight away add all of it to the mortar and it should be triturated in one direction until the mixture becomes thick and the primary emulsion is made. The primary emulsion is characterized by a clicking sound.
3. Calculate the unused vehicle.
4. Divide the unused vehicle into three parts: 1- For dilution of the primary emulsion, 2-For washing the mortar and pestle, and 3-For completing the emulsion to its final volume.

v. Wet Gum Method

1. Water is added to the acacia gum and quickly triturated until the gum dissolves, to make mucilage.
2. Oil is added to this mucilage in small portions drop by drop, triturating the mixture thoroughly after each addition until a thick primary emulsion is formed.
3. Then dilute the primary emulsion with small volumes of the vehicle.
4. Then add any other ingredient.

6. Transfer to a measuring cylinder and makeup to final volume with the vehicle.

Differences between wet and dry gum methods:

•Emulsifying agents are mixed with the oil in the dry gum method and it is mixed with water in the wet gum method.

•Addition of water will be all at once in the dry gum method, while the oil is added drop by drop in the wet method.

• The crackling sound is heard higher in the wet method than in the dry method.

2. Bottle Method [Forbes Bottle Method]

The bottle method is convenient for the formulation of emulsions from volatile oil or oleaginous substances of low viscosity. Powdered acacia is placed in a dry bottle, two parts of oil are added, and the mixtures are shaken in the closed container. A volume of water approximately equal to that of the oils are then added in portions and the mixture is properly shaken after each addition. When all of the water has been added then the primary emulsion thus formed may be diluted to the proper volume with water. This method is not suited for the viscous oils because they cannot be simply agitated in the bottle when mixed with the emulsifying agents.

Stability Problems of Emulsion

Emulsions are colloid mixtures prepared by mixing two unmixable liquids, usually oil and water, which liquefy into one of the liquids. Emulsion have two phases. The first phase is of particles, and the second is the liquid surrounding particles.

FACTORS AFFECTING THE STABILITY OF AN EMULSIONs:

- Increased particle size of the internal phase causes the decrease in the stability of an emulsion. So, smaller size of the particles of the internal phase is always selected.
- Deflocculated particles are always selected because if there is less particle-particle interaction there will be more stability of an emulsion
- For more stability there should be less particle density

- Bulk phase/external phase density - For more stability of an emulsion, there should be more bulk phase density
- The more the viscosity of bulk phase the more the stability of the emulsion

Instability of an emulsions and Methods to overcome

Flocculations:

Flocculations are the joining together of globules to form large floccules inside the emulsion in flocculation the interfacial film and the individual droplets remain intact the globules do not coalesce and by agitating it will be redispersed.

Remedy

The presence of high charged density on the distributed droplet will check the presence of a high energy barrier and then reduce the occurrence of flocculation

Creaming:

Creaming is the mixing or setting of distributed globules to make a concentrated layer at the bottom of the emulsion.

Remedy:

1. Reduction of the globules by utilizing a high systematic homogenizer.
2. Increasing the viscosity of the continuous phase by utilizing the viscosity imparting agent
3. By decreasing the density difference between two phases
4. By managing the dispersed phase concentration
5. By storing it in a cool place or at low temperature.

Coalescence:

Coalescence is agitated of the drops into larger drops. In coalescence, the droplet loses their individuality. During the interfacial film is demolished. So, coalescence is irreversible. Droplets cannot be redistributed by agitating.

Remedy

1. By adding a required amount of emulsifying agents and passing the product through the required emulsifying machinery.
2. During formulations the addition of emulsifying agents should be appropriate because using the wrong emulsifying agent it will loses their activity in short period of time.

Breaking or Cracking:

Cracking means the disassociation of two layers of dispersing and continuous phase, Due to the coalescence of distributed phase globules which are difficult to re-distribute

THE CRACKING IS DUE TO THE FOLLOWING: -

(1) Addition of emulsifying agents of the opposite type

(2) Decayed or precipitation of emulgent

(3) Common solvent is added.

(4) Microorganisms

(5) Temperature change

Pharmaceutical Applications of emulsions

•Emulsions (macroemulsions and micro emulsions) are generally well registered as water loving and lipid loving drug carriers.

•Oils and drugs having unpleasant taste or texture can be made more palatable for oral administration by preparing it into emulsions.

•On topically applied emulsion, the formulation scientist can control cosmetic and dermatologic products' viscosity, appearance, and degree of greasiness. O/W emulsions are most convenient as water-washable bases, whereas water-in-oil (w/o) emulsions are used for treating dry skin and emollient applications to provide an occlusive effect.

•Semisolid formulations, such as creams and ointments, represent the distribution of liquids in solids, which are used in topical application.

Model questions

- Define and classify emulsion.
- What is emulsifying agents? Give mechanism of emulsifying agents.
- Give theories of emulsification.
- Explain different identification tests for emulsion.
- Explain different methods of preparation of emulsion.
- How emulsion stability is assessed? Explain different remedies for instability of emulsion.
- Elaborate different stability problems in emulsion.
- Write a note on:

(1) Multiple emulsion
(ii) Nano-emulsion
(ii) Emulsifying agents
(iii) Microemulsions

CHAPTER XI

Suppositories

INTRODUCTION

Suppositories are solid dosage forms intended for insertion in to body cavities or orifices other than mouth (Rectum, Vagina & Urethra).

Suppositories are designed to either melt or dissolve in the cavity fluids after insertion, releasing the medication and having a regional or therapeutic effect on the body.

The word "suppositories" is derived from the Latin "Suppositorium," which meaning "to place under." Suppositories have been used to provide medication to elderly individuals and other patients who were unable to do so through more conventional routes. When inserted, suppositories act as a protector or a palliative for the local tissue. And also transport medications for systemic or local use.

Suppositories typically consist of an active medication mixed into a base that is either rigid or semi-rigid and an inert matrix. There shouldn't be any interactions between the medicine and the inert matrix. Suppository bases carry, protect, and deliver active medication to patients while dispersing or diluting it. After being delivered, suppositories melt at body temperature and release the medication by dissolving in mucosal fluids, where the active ingredient first manifests its local effects before manifesting its systemic effects after being transported to the bloodstream. The both non- clinical and clinical performance of suppositories are significantly influenced by the physi - cochemical qualities of both the medication and suppository bases.

Suppositories come in a variety of sizes, shapes, volumes, and consistency that make it easier for them to be inserted and retained in the cavity.

Suppositories' indications :

The following situations call for the usage of suppositories:

(i) To clear the bowels prior to specific surgeries.

(ii) To ease acute constipation or when other constipation therapies haven't worked.

(iii) To evacuate the bowels before to an endoscopic examination .

(iv) To administer medication to the body.

(v) Hemorrhoids or anal pruritus can be treated or soothed in this way .

Indications against using suppositories

Suppositories should not be used if one or more of the following apply:

(i) Chronic constipation that would necessitate frequent use.

(ii) Ileus paralysis.

(iii) Colonic blockage

(iv) After gynaecological or digestive operations, unless under a doctor's explicit orders.

- **Classification of suppositories:**

There are 5 types of suppositories according to the route of administration

1. Rectal suppositories
2. Vaginal suppositories
3. Urethral suppositories
4. Nasal suppositories
5. Ear suppositories

1. **Rectal suppositorie**

To provide a therapeutic impact, these are designed for injection into the rectum.

Rectal suppositories often have a broader midsection before tapering towards the other end, which helps with retention in the rectum and makes it possible for the anal sphincter to push the suppository forward.

Adult rectal suppositories typically weigh 2 gm and however paediatric suppositories are substantially smaller in size than adult suppositories. Suppositories for kids typically weigh approximately 1 gm.

They treat ailments such:

a) costiveness also known as constipation;

b) hyperthermia also known as fever;

c) haemorrhoids;

d) mental health illnesses like schizophrenia, anxiety, or bipolar disorder; and

e) nausea, especially motion sickness.

f) ache

Examples;

a. Paracetamol 1.P. 80 mg, 170 mg, or 250 mg: Antipyretic; Suppol® Baby/Child/250 (Meridian);
b. GV-SOFT (Bliss) 2. 90% w/w Glycerin USP: Laxative
c. Sun Pharma's Mesacol® Suppositories: For the treatment of the intestinal condition ulcerative proctitis, mesalamine 500 mg is used.

2. Vaginal suppositories:

Vaginal suppositories are often referred to as Pessaries.Pessaries are solid pharmaceutical preparations that are designed to be inserted into the vagina for either local or systemic action.

Pessaries can weigh anything between 3 and 5 g, hence a larger mould is needed for them than for rectal suppositories. They come in globular, oviform, rod, wedge, compressed on a tablet press into conical shapes (vaginal tablets), as well as capsule and capsule-like forms (vaginal capsule).

Pessaries can be placed into the vagina with your fingers, however applicators are available for pessaries with unique shapes to make the process easier. Except for a few drugs, like prostaglandin, which have an impact throughout the body, pessaries are only utilised for their local activity in the vagina.

Antiseptics, contraceptives, local anaesthetics, and other therapeutic medications to treat trichomonal, bacterial, and mononuclear infections are often used drugs for inclusion in pessaries.

Uses for pessaries / vaginal suppositories : Before using pessaries, wash your hands and read the medicine package. the pessary and applicator of any foil or plastic packing (if supplied). Put the pessary in the hole at the end of the applicator, if one is provided. With your legs wide and your knees bent, sit or lie down. Using either fingers or the applicator, gently introduce the pessary as far into the vagina as is comfortable. In the event that an applicator is being utilised, depress the plunger to release the pessary before removing it from the vagina. Rewash your hands.

Examples:

1. Glenmark's Candid CL® Vaginal Pessary, 200 mg of clotrimazole and 100 mg of clindamycin.
2. TODAY® Vaginal Contraceptive (Bliss GVS); Vaginal Contraceptive: Nonoxynol -9 USP-5%w/w.
3. Novo Nordisk's Vagifem Estradiol Vaginal Tablets: Estradiol 10 mcg: Used to treat vaginal abnormalities brought on by menopause.

3. Urethral suppositories:

The urethral suppositories are intended for urethral insertion.

The female urethral suppositories weigh 2 gm a piece, while the male urethral suppositorie weigh 4 gm a peice & measure 100-150 mm in length.

These have a pencil-like form and are also known as urethral bougies.

In rare instances, men may use a specific kind of urethral suppository to treat erection issues.

Alprostadil, a medication, is delivered by these rice-grain-sized suppositories.

Example;

For urethral suppository MUSE® (Alprostadil) : to treat erectile dysfunction can use 125 mcg of alprostadil .

4. Nasal suppositories:

The purpose of the nasal suppositories is to be introduced into the nasal cavity.

They are often made with base of glycerogelatin. They are shaped similarly to the Urinary bougies They are approximately 1 gramme in weight and 9–10 cm long.

Nasal bougies or buginaria are other names for nasal suppositories.

5. Ear cones:

These devices are inserted into the ear. These are rarely employed. The base used to prepare ear cones is generally Theobroma oil. These are also known as Aurinaria

Other Special Type of Suppositories:

1. **Tablet Suppositories:**

- These suppositories are prepare by compression method same as in tablet compression.
- It is utilised for both vaginal and rectal routes.
- There are two almond-shaped Pessaries tablet suppositories in the package.
- Rectal tablets with protective thin coatings of components like polyethylene glycol.
- Since these tablet suppositories are made with super disintegrants and dissolve in the presence of low fluid levels in the body cavity, it is not required to store them at lower temperatures. Polyethylene glycol (PEG) is typically coated on tablet suppositories to protect them and make it easier to inject them into the rectum.

1. **Layered Suppositories:**

- Layered suppositories are made with different drugs in different layers to avoid incompatibility between those drugs.
- Drugs with various melting points can also be added to modulate the rate of absorption.
- It can be made by partially filling a mould with a drug and base matrix, then after it has solidified or congealed, filling the mould with a separate layer of a different drug and base matrix.

3. **Coated Suppositories**

- Coated suppositories made with free unsaturated fatty acids, polyethylene glycol, etc. for their smooth lubricating properties.
- These materials have lubricating qualities that restrict their rate of disintegration and offer storage protection.

4. **Capsule Suppositories**

- These types of suppositories are manufactured with soft gelatin capsules in a variety of sizes & shapes.
- Liquids, semisolids, or solids can be found inside capsule suppositories. The popularity of these capsules is rising.

5. **Packaging in disposable moulds:**

- These days, suppositories are created directly in disposable plastic or tin foil moulds rather than metallic ones, where the latter require individual packaging and delivery in boxes.
- The benefit of this kind of suppository is that, in the event that the contents melt for whatever reason while being transported or stored, they will still be in the mould and can be used after chilling in the refrigerator.

6. **Hollow-Type Suppositories:**

- These suppositories have a hollow hole to accommodate different drug dosages, such as a powder or solution. As opposed to conventional suppository, it is thought to be superior because it is not impacted by the qualities of the base.

- Drugs are released from hollow suppositories more quickly than they are from regular suppositories.

7. **Hydrogel Suppositories:**

- The term "hydrogel" refers to the macromolecular network employed as the base in this form of suppository that swells but does not dissolve in water.
- The amount and rate of drug release from this hydrogel matrix depends on the rate of drug diffusion out of the swollen matrix and the migration of water into the matrix.

8. **Sectile or Bisected Suppositories:**

- Suppositories with a bisected or bevelled edge in the centre are referred to as sectile or bisected suppositories. The middle of the suppository is divided so that a youngster can use half of it after being sliced, and an adult can use the entire thing.

9. **Sustained Release Suppositories:**

- These suppositories are designed to delay medication release from the base for a longer period of time, hence reducing the need for repeated administrations and maintaining therapeutic impact.

10. **Thermo-Reversible-Liquid Suppository:**

- At body temperature, these liquid suppositories turn into gel. It contains adequate gel strength so that after administration, it won't leak out of the anus.
- Such a gel won't reach the end of the colon since it lacks the necessary mucoadhesive power.

11. **Effervescent Suppository:**

- The suppository base in this type of suppository contains a mixture of citric or tartaric acid and sodium bicarbonate.
- Following administration, fluid absorption results in effervescence, which breaks down the suppository and releases the drug.

ADVANTAGES OF SUPPOSITORIES:-

1. Suppository allows for self-administration.
2. It can be used to circumvent first-pass metabolism and allow for systemic medication absorption.
3. It can influence the rectal mucosa locally.
4. It safeguards the medicine against harsh stomach conditions.
5. It prevents any drug-related stomach discomfort.
6. The drug, which can be delivered using suppositories, produces nausea and vomiting.
7. Suppository usage is practical before surgery when oral intake is prohibited.
8. It is practical for post-operative patients who cannot be given oral medication.
9. Patients with severe vomiting and those who are unconscious can use it (for example, during fitting).
10. It has a large capacity for drug loading.

11. Suppository use may be used for lymphatic delivery.

12. It gives the environment for medication absorption a steady and unchanging state.

13. The medication has a speedier onset of action than after oral administration since it is directly absorbed from the mucosa into the venous circulation.

14. It can be applied to a distribution system that is site-specific.

DISADVANTAGES OF SUPPOSITORIES:-

1. Irritant drug can not be administered
2. Embarrassing to some patients
3. Need to be store at low temp.
4. Can't be easily prepared
5. Cost-expensive.
6. The rectum has a considerably lower fluid level than the small intestine; that could affect things like dissolving rate and other things.
7. The microbial flora found in the rectum may breakdown some drugs.
8. **Variables influencing medication absorption from a suppository:-**

A. **Physiological Factors:-**

(1) Fluid availability: There is relatively little fluid available for medication dispersion (approximately 3 mL). As a result, the absorption process' slowest step is the dissolution of marginally soluble compounds.

(ii) Rectal fluid characteristics: The fluid has a pH of 7-8 neutrality and no buffering ability.

(iii) The rectum's contents : When desired systemic effects are needed, greater absorption from an empty rectum may be predicted because the drug will be in close contact with the rectum's absorbent surface.

(iv) Route of circulation: Medicine is absorbed and begins to circulate throughout the body without going via the liver in the lower hemorrhoidal veins that surround the colon. The lymphatic system helps in absorption as well.

B. **Drug and suppository basis physicochemical characteristics**

The relative solubility of a drug in lipid and in water, as well as its particle size, pka, dose, and other physical and chemical characteristics, as well as the suppository base's ability to release the therapeutic material, melted, soft , and dissolve at body temperature, and possess either hydrophilic or hydrophobic qualities all have an impact on how well a drug is absorbed through the suppository.

(i)Drug solubility in vehicle: The solubility of medication in the vehicle, or moe specifically, its partition coefficient between the vehicle and the rectal liquid, directly affects how quickly it is released from a suppository and absorbed by the rectal mucous membrane. The likelihood for medications to leave the vehicle will be minimal when they are highly soluble in the vehicle, which will result in a low release rate into the rectal fluid.

(ii) Particle Size: The size of the drug particle will affect the rate of dissolution and the amount of drug that is available for absorption for medications that are present in a suppository in the undissolved condition. The likelihood of quick absorption increases with decreasing particle size and increased ease of breakdown.

(iii) Base nature :.To release the drug's component parts for absorption, the base's nature must able to melt, soft , and dissolve. Medication absorptions will be hampered and even blocked if the base interacts with the drug to limit its release. The base may cause a colonic reaction and a bowel movement if it irritates the mucous membranes of the rectum, which could result in insufficient medication release and absorption.

(iv) Spreading Capacity: The extent to which the melted base: drug mixture covers the surface area of the rectal mucous membrane determines the speed and potency of the therapeutic effects of suppositories (the spreading capacity of the suppositories). The presence of surfactants in the base may be responsible for this spreading potential.

- **Suppository uses include:**

The primary uses of suppositories are for their mechanical, localised, and systemic actions.

i. In the treatment of haemorrhoids, anal irritation, and constipation, suppositories are used to get mechanical action to assist bowel evacuation by irritating the mucous membrane of the rectum or by lubricating action.
ii. Suppository can be used for local action for drugs like emollients, astringents, antisept local anaesthetics, and antibiotics, among others.
iii. Drugs that have a systemic effect include analgesics, antispasmodics, sedatives, hypnotics, tranquillizers, vasodilators, hormones, etc.

FORMULATION OF SUPPOSITORY :-

For formulation of suppository following components are required .

a. Drug (active pharmaceutical ingredient)
b. Suppository base
c. Additives
d. Packaging material

a) Drug (Active Pharmaceutical Ingredient) :-

Drugs with GIT stability issues or medications that irritate the stomach mucosa can be used to make suppositories. Drugs that are prescribed to treat problems of the lower colon may be used in the preparation of suppositories.

Suppository-form medications can be produced for use in comatose and treatment of pregnancy, chemotherapy, and allergy-induced emesis in paediatric patients, as well as . Suppositories are made from medications that require sustained-release for the long-term management of chronic conditions as essential hypertension, asthma, diabetes, AIDS, anaemia, etc.

To generate a lighter suppository, the drug to be put into it should have a minimal basis. To achieve homogeneity, a drug must be soluble in a base, but it must not lower the base's melting point. During preparation and use, it should be stable and compatible with the suppository's base and other additives.

(b) **SUPPOSITORY BASES :-**

Drugs are carried by suppository bases, which also dilute the medication to make it less irritating and control how much of the drug is released from the suppository. To aid or promote the release of the drug in such a way that it is readily available for absorption, the suppository base must melt, soften, or dissolve.

Drug stability and bioavailability may be impacted by physico-chemical interactions with the suppository bases; as a result, such potential interactions must be investigated in preformulation studies. If the base of a suppository irritates the mucous membrane, it will trigger a colonic response and so encourage an undesirable somatic reaction that could result in the expulsion of the dose form and impair drug absorption.

Ideal Properties of Suppositories Bases

1.It ought to not be poisonous, irritable, or sensitive to inflamed tissue.

2.At the temperature of the rectal cavity (36°C) or any other body cavity, it should melt.

3.It shouldn't have a meta-stable form and should be compatible with additives and medications.

4.It should be able to assimilate more water (should have a high "water number")

5.It should have sufficient volume contraction upon cooling for easy release from moulds.

6.It need to have emulsifying and wetting qualities.

7.Over the course of storage, it should remain physically and chemically stable (shelf-life)

8.Iodine value should be less than 7, acid value should be less than 0.2, and saponification value should be between 200 and 245.

9.The solid fat index (SFI), or the distance between the melting and solidification points, should be narrow.

10.When stored on a shelf, the suppository base should be high viscosity at low shear and low viscosity at high shearing rates (agitation pouring and spreading). Thus, thixotropic and pseudoplastic bases are advantageous because they solidify when left alone and liquefy when disturbed.

11.Both easily and cheaply accessible.

- The suppository should have all of the aforementioned desirable features because it must maintain its shape, stiffness, and firmness throughout administration and storage but should melt inside the human cavity.
- However, it is challenging to obtain all desirable features from a single base; as a result, combinations of various suppository bases are frequently utilised to obtain desired suppository properties.

Types of Suppositories Bases:-

Oleaginous (fatty) bases that dissolve or spread in rectal secretion and water soluble or kater miscible bases that melt at body temperature are of two different types of suppository bases that can be categorised based on their composition and physical properties.

Suppository bases are classified into two major categories

1. Fatty suppository bases – they are designed to melt at body temperature
2. Hydrophilic Suppository base
3. water - miscible bases – they will scatter or dissolve in rectal secretion
4. Emulsifying base : which help a small amount of drug's aqueous solution to emulsify.

Fatty Base

1. Cocoa butter / Theobroma oil

2.Emulsified theobroma oil

3. Shea butter

4.Hydrogenated bases.

1.Theobroma oil/ Cocoa butter :-

It is a solid that is yellowish-white in colour and tastes and smells like chocolate.

It consists of a mixture of stearic, palmitic, oleic, and other unsaturated fatty acid glyceryl esters.

Its melting point is between 30 and 35 °C, so overheating alters its physical properties, and when hardened, it has a propensity to stick to the mould.

The iodine content is between 34 and 38.

Because cocoa butter might melt and go rancid, its acid value should not be greater than 4. As a result, it must be kept in a dry, cold environment and away from light.

Theobroma oil may exist in four crystalline states:-

a. **α** : The melted substance is abruptly cooled to 0°C to produce this form. It has a 24 °C melting point.
b. **β**: When cocoa butter is slowly melted at 35 to 36°C, and cooled slowly it takes on the β Form. At 18 to 23 °C, it melts.**β`**: It returns to the three forms in the β form and melts about 34 to 35°C.
c. ϒ: It is made by adding a container with chilled (20°C) cocoa butter before it is chilled to a deep freeze temperature before solidifying. At 18 °C, it melts.

Cocoa butter should be melted and cooled with extreme caution. As is usually the case, it is advised to use as little heat as possible during melting.

Advantages of Theobroma oil :-

(a) Has a melting point range of 30 to 36 °C; hence, it is solid at standard room temperatures but melts when consumed.

(b) Rapid setting upon cooling and ready liquefaction upon reheating.

(c) Miscibility with a variety of substances.

(d) Boringness, or the absence of irritation

Disadvantage of Theobroma oil:-

(1).Polymorphism: Three polymorphs of cocoa butter exist: α -crystals, which are unstable at 20°C, β - crystals, which are stable at 36°C, and ϒ-crystals, which are unstable at 15°C.

Depending on the melting temperature, velocity of cooling, and mass size, it solidifies upon melting and cooling in various crystalline shapes.

It produces stable -crystals with a normal melting point when melted below 36°C and slowly cooled, but if overheated, it may produce unstable -crystals that melt at approximately 15°C or -crystals that melt at about 20°C. It may take many days for these unstable forms to recover to their stable state, during which time the suppositories may not set at room temperature or, if set by cooling, may remelt in the patient's home's heat.

The solidification point being lowered may also cause suspended solids to settle out. Consequently, when producing theobroma oil suppositories, extreme caution must be used to prevent overheating the base.

(2) Adherence to mould: Sticking may happen, especially if the mould is worn, since theobroma oil does not compress enough upon cooling to free the suppositories in the mould. By lubricating the mould before usage, this is avoided.

(3) Low softening point for hot climates: Theobroma oil suppositories made for usage in tropical and subtropical regions might have white beeswax added to them to enhance the softening point.

(4) Melting point reduced by soluble ingredients : Theobroma oil's melting point may be significantly lowered by substances that dissolve in it, such as chloral hydrate, making the suppositories too pliable to be used. A regulated amount of white beeswax may be applied to raise the melting point.

(5) Slow deterioration during storage: The unsaturated glycerides oxidise, causing this.

(6) A lack of ability to absorb water: Emulsifying chemicals can help with this flaw.

(7) Body leakage: The rectum or vagina might occasionally let molten base out. Due to their increased size and the difficulty this causes, theobroma oil is rarely used to make pessaries.

(8) fairly high price : Emulsified theobroma oil, hydrogenated palm kernel oil, and soyabean oil have all been proposed as alternatives to cocoa butter to address its shortcomings.

2.Emulsified Theobroma Oil:

This emulsifiy theobroma oil is use as a basis when a substantial amount of water solution have to added to a suppository in order to encourage the diffusion of the active medicinal ingredient to the surrounding tissue and its subsequent absorption.

It is made by emulsifying theobroma oil with various emulsifying agents; for instance, adding 5% glyceryl monostearate will result in a product with a 35°C melting point that can be used as the basis for either a hot or cold suppository preparation procedure.

An oil-in-water emulsified basis is created using 2% lecithin and 98% theobroma oil. Theobroma oil and 2% cholesterol will result in a water-in-oil emulsion.

Other ingredients used to create emulsified theobroma oil include up to 12% spermaceti wax, 4% bees wax, 2-3% cetyl alcohol, and 10% lanette wax.

3.Shea butter :-

From the seeds of the Sapotaceae family's shea tree, Butyrospermum parkii, shea butter has been produced.

It contains 46-59% oleic acid and 36-44% glycerides of stearic acid.

It is compatible with several medications and has a melting point of 37.8°C.

It can absorb water well. It can be utilised to enhance the physicochemical and drug release qualities combined with polysorbate 80 and beeswax.

4.Hydrogenated Oils (Also known as Synthetic fats bases):-

A number of hydrogenated oils, such as hydrogenated edible oil, arachis oil, coconut oil, palm kernel oil, stearic and a combination of oleic and stearic acids are suggested as theobroma oil substitutes.

Vegetable oils like palm oil and arachis oil are hydrogenated and then heated to create the bases for synthetic suppositories. In most cases, the oils are esters of unsaturated fatty acids.

Unsaturated fatty acids are saturated by hydrogenation, and heat treatment breaks up certain triglycerides into fatty acids and partial esters (mono and di-glycerides).

Advantages of these synthetic fats over theobroma oil:

1. Overheating does not influence their solidifying points.
2. Due to the reduction of their unsaturated fatty acids, they exhibit good resistance to oxidation.
3. They have high emulsifying and water-absorbing abilities. They typically contain a percentage of partial glycerides, some of which, like glyceryl monostearate, do not contain emulsifying agents, therefore they have high emulsifying and water absorption properties.
4. Due to their substantial cooling-induced contraction, no mould lubricant is necessary.
5. They create tasteful, odourless, and colourless suppositories.
6. There is little distinction between melting and setting points. So they immediately set. There is little chance that substances in suspension will settle.
7. They can be chosen from a range of grades with varying melting points that are available for sale to suit certain products and environmental conditions.

Disadvantages:

1.They shouldn't be chilled because if they are, they will become brittle. A few chemicals, including polysorbate 80 at 0.05%, can help to fix this flaw.

2. When melted, they are more fluid than theobroma oil and the rate of sedimentation is higher. To lessen this, thickeners like colloidal silicon dioxide, bentonite, and magnesium stearate may be used.

Hydrophilic Suppository base :-

1. Water-soluble / water miscible bases :-

(a) Glycerol -Gelatine base

The inclusion of gelatine thickens and stiffens the glycerol - gelatine base , which is a mixture of glycerine and water. Since glycerol gelatine base is hydrophilic by nature, suppositories made with it give a slow, continuous release of medication by slowly dissolving in aqueous secretions.

All different kinds of suppositories can be made with it, but vaginal suppositories benefit the most from its use.

Solid extracts, such as belladonna, can be added to it with ease. It can also be used for medications including opium, bromides, chloral hydrate, iodide, and iodoform, as well as suppositories containing boric acid.

For their efficient usage as antiseptics, glycerol gelatine basis is also advised for products like hexyl resorcinol, nitromersol , and phemeral in suppository form.

Ingredient	**BP and IP**	**USP**	**BPC**
Gelatine	14g	20g	25g
Glycerine	70g	70g	40g
Water to	100g	100g	100g
	For solid drugs and liquids < 20 %		For liquid > 20%

The composition of glycerol gelatine base as per different pharmacopeia is:-

As a foundation for suppositories, two forms of gelatin are employed.

(i) Type-A or Pharmagel- A: which is made by acid hydrolysis (has isoelectric point between 7 to 9 and on the acid side of the range behaves as a cationic agent, being most effective at pH 7 to 8.) is used for acidic drugs.

(ii) Type B or Pharmagel- B: which is prepared by alkaline hydrolysis (having an isoelectric point between 4.7 to 5 and on the alkaline side of the range behaves as an anionic agent, being most effective at pH 7 to 8) is used for alkaline drugs

Disadvantages

Glycero gelain base suppositories are less commonly used than the fatty base suppositories because:

i. They had laxative action.

ii. They require greater preparation time and more management.

iii. The amount of gelatin present, its calibre, and the base's age all affect how quickly they dissolve.

iv. Drugs that precipitate with the protein, such as tannic acid, ferric chloride, gallic acid, etc., are incompatible with gelatin.

v. Osmosis, a physiological process that results in a laxative effect, happens during the process of dissolving in the mucous secretions of the rectum.

Vi .lubricating the mould is important

vii. Because there is only a less amount of liquid present, it may induce rectal irritation.

viii.Unpredictable solution time

ix. Hygroscopic: They should be packaged in airtight containers since they dehydrate the vaginal and rectal mucosa, which might irritate them.

x. probability of microbial contamination is more.

xi. take longer time for preparation.

(b) Soap – Glycerin Suppositories :-

• In this situation, a significant amount of glycerin—up to 95% of the mass—can be added, along with gelatin, curd soap, or sodium stearate, which renders the glycerin sufficiently hard for suppositories.

The downside of soap glycerin suppositories is that they are extremely hygroscopic, therefore they must be shielded from the atmosphere and covered in waxed paper or tin foil.

Moreover, the soap aids in the evacuation of glycerin.

(c) Polyethylene glycol bases:-

Polyethylene glycol's International Non-proprietary Name (INN) is macrogol (PEG). They are ethylene oxide, water, and their ether-based polymers.

It goes by the names "carbowaxes" and "polyglycols." PEG with a molecular weight between 200 and 1000 has a liquid consistency, while PEG with a molecular weight over 1000 has a waxy consistency.

With increasing molecular weight, their water solubility, hygroscopicity, and vapour pressure decrease.

Combining different molecular weights of PEG allows for the creation of suppositories with various melting points.

The following mixtures are typically used to prepare suppositories:

COMPOSITION OF PEG	USE
PEG 1000 – 96% PEG 4000 – 04%	This base is soft and used for fast release of drug.
PEG 1000 – 75% PEG 4000- 25%	It is used for slow release of drug.
PEG 1540 – 70% PEG 6000 – 30%	It is used for drug having lower melting point.
PEG 1540 – 30 % PEG 6000 – 50% WATER – 20%	As it contains water, it is used for water soluble drugs.

Advantages:

(i) Chemically inert (no laxative effect) and physiologically inert

(ii) No need for lubricant during moulding stableas base compresses somewhat.

(iii) There is less microbial contamination.

(iv)Has the potential for both instant and extended effect.

(v)Cool storage is not necessary because the melting point is above body temperature (42°C); (vi) It has good solvent properties.

(vii) Create suppository that looks tidy and smooth.

(vii) Because of their large molecular weight, high viscosity solutions are created when substances disperse throughout the body, and leaking is not a major issue.

Disadvatages:-

(i) Hygroscopic, therefore it needs special storage conditions and could dry up and irritate the rectum.

(ii) Compatibility problems, Several medications, such phenols and tannins, cannot be used with polyethylene glycol bases. Additionally, some antibacterial agents, like hydroxy benzoate and quaternary ammonium compounds, lose some of their antibacterial action. They also affect various polymers, which restricts the available container options.

(iii) Diminished therapeutic impact: Drug retention in the liquefied base due to good solvent characteristics can have a reduced therapeutic effect.

(iv)The result could be brittle suppository.

2. Emulsifying Bases:-

- These bases are synthetic, and other high-quality proprietary bases are also offered.
- Emulsifying bases are sold under the trade names Massa Esterinum , Witepsol, and Massupol.

(a) Witepsol :

It is a white, odourless base made up of different ratios of partial esters in triglycerides of saturated vegetal acids. Additionally included is the beeswax for usage in hot conditions. There are nine grades available, however the most commonly used ones are Witepsol He Hs. Was Sss Ers and Ess. They are ideal for the formulation of tropical suppositories and eutectic matures. Witepsol-prepared suppositories shouldn't be ice-cooled or allowed to cool quickly because doing so could cause them to crack. Additionally, while using this foundation, mould must not be greased. When heated and cooled, it has no polymorphisms.

(b) Massa Esterium: .

Its other name is Adeps solidus. It is a mixture of saturated fatty acid monoglycerides, diglycerides, and triglycerides with the chemical formula C11H23COOH to C17H35COOH.

There are various Mass estrinum grades, including Massaestrinum A AB, AS, B, BB, BC, BD, and C.

It is a solid that is white, brittle, practically flavourless, and odourless. Their melting point ranges from 33 to 38 °C.

(c) Massuppol:

It is mostly made up of glyceryl esters of lauric acid, with a little quantity of glyceryl monostearate added to increase its ability to absorb water..

It can be mass produced and has a melting range of 34 to 37°C.

All of these bases are devoid of the negative effects of cocoa butter and don't need to be lubricated against mould.

Surfactants are essentially what make up water-dispersible bases. At body temperature, they dissolve. Below is a list of some dispersible base formulas that contain surfactants. 10 glyceryl monostearate, 15 glyceryl monostearate, 60,40 tween

(d) Wecobee bases:-

It is made from triglycerides of coconut oil and palm kernel oil's higher melting fractions, and it may contain 0.25% lecithin. They become emulsifiable when glyceryl monostearate and propylene glycol monostearate are added.

(e) Dehydarz bases

This foundation comes in three grades: L, II, and G. These grades can be used to create suppository. Hardened fatty alcohols and lipids are present in grades I and II, and saturated fatty alcohol is present in grade G. Wax or high melting alcohols may be added to raise the melting point of grade I and II. There is no polymorphism present.

Advantages over cocoa butter of these bases

1. Excessive heating does not change the physical properties.
2. They are not mold-stickable. They don't need the mould to be previously lubricated.
3. They quickly solidify.
4. They have a lower risk of going rancid.
5. They have a sizable capacity for aqueous liquid absorption.

Dsadvantages;

1)Because they are not very viscous, other medications may settle down.

2) When refrigerated or immediately after a rapid chilling, they become brittle.

Additives

Suppositories are made softer and more resilient by the use of plasticizers such cetyl alcohol and propylene glycol. In order to promote the absorption of drugs with low bioavailability, such as antibiotics, and high molecular weights, absorption-promoting compounds are also employed as an addition in suppositories. Antioxidants (such BHA and BHT) are additional additives that are employed based on need and only after being tested for compatibility with the medicine and suppository base.

Packeging Materials:-

1. Blister packaging: PVC film is typically utilised as a kind of packaging, while aluminium foil may also be employed depending on the situation. The blister pack typically contains 5 suppositories, and those blisters are then put into a carton with 2 blisters each.

2. Strip Packing: Pouch-style strips made of four layers of material (poly, aluminium, poly, and paper, with poly as the inner layer and paper as the exterior layer) that each contain five suppositories. These strips are then placed in a carton with 2 strips per strip,
3. Bottle packing: Plastic bottles sealed with aluminium taggers. Such bottles are then further packaged in a bottle-containing e-flute carton. Finally, these e-flute boxes are placed into a master corrugated shipper.
4. Plastic disposable moulds: Suppositories are now often packaged in plastic that can be thrown away. The benefit of this type of packaging is that if the suppository liquefies while being transported or stored, the contents will still be contained in the plastic disposable mould and can still be used after being refrigerated.

STRATEGIES FOR PREPARATION:-

One of three procedures can be used to produce suppositories:-

1.Hand Rolling:-

When only a small number of suppositories need to be manufactured in a cocoa butter base, this is the easiest and oldest way of preparing suppositories. It has the benefit of not requiring to heat the cocoa butter.

A plastic-like material is created by triturating active substances and cocoa butter that has been grated in a mortar. After being formed into a ball in the palm of the hands, the material is first rolled into a consistent cylinder using a large spatula or a small flat board on a pill tile.. After being chopped into the necessary number of parts, the cylinder is subsequently rolled on to create a conical form at one end.

Particularly when the bulk is not thoroughly kneaded and softened, the suppository "pipe" or cylinder frequently cracks or becomes hollow in the middle.

2.Compression Molding:-

Compression moulding is a technique for making suppositories by forcing a mixture of grated suppository base and medications into a specialised compression mould using suppository manufacturing equipment. The additional ingredients are well mixed with the suppository foundation. Because of the friction created throughout the process, the base softens. For small scale, you can use a mortar and pestle. On the other hand, large-scale manufacturing uses warmed mixing vessels and mechanically driven kneading mixers. The suppository material is inserted into a cylinder and then sealed inside the compression machine. The bulk is then released from the other end into the suppository mould or die by applying pressure from one end. A moveable end plate at the back of the die is removed once the die is filled with the mass, and the produced suppositories are expelled when further pressure is applied to the bulk in the cylinder.. When all of the suppository mass has been used, the end plate is brought back and the procedure is repeated. Based on the density considerations, it is important to omit some of the suppository foundation when the active components are applied one of the active components.

3.Fusion Molding:-

In order to prevent overheating, the suppository base is first melted on a water bath before the medication is either emulsified or suspended in it during the heated process.

Then, this mass is put to a suppository mould that has been previously greased, where it is allowed to cool.

In both the laboratory and the industrial setting, it is a commonly utilised technique for making suppository.

4. Suppository Moulds:-

The suppository mould is comprised of brass, aluminium, nickel-copper alloy, and stainless steel. It has 6-12 cavities that are the right size and form. It is possible to use a mould with 500 cavities for large-scale production. Industrial moulds produce thousands of suppositories per hour from a single moulding.

Calibration of the Mould

The calibration of the mould is required because, while the size of the suppositories produced by a given mould is constant, their weight fluctuates due to the disparity in base and medication densities. Making moulded suppositories solely out of base material is the initial stage. The average weight of the suppositories is calculated. The volume of the melt is determined to determine the size of the mould after the suppositories are melted in a calibrated beaker.

Lubrication use in moulds:-

For mould lubrication, glycero-gelatine bases and cocoa butter are needed. This helps to avoid bases clinging to the mould cavity wall. Additionally, it helps with the simple removal of suppositories from the moulds. The lubricants create a coating between the base of the suppositories and the wall of the mould chamber, preventing the bases from sticking to the moulds. Lubricants should have a different nature from bases.

Lubricant needs to be compatible with any adjuncts or medications. Silicone fluid is used as lubricant in industries. A thin, reasonably stiff brush or a pad of muslin or gauze are used to lubricate the mould. Since certain cotton wool fibres stick to the mould, cotton wool is not used. By turning the mould on a clean white tile, extra lubricant can be eliminated.

Theobroma oil suppositories may be made using the following lubricants.

Examples:

(a)For bases made of cocoa butter.

50 ml alcohol (90%)

10 ml of glycerol

10 grams of soft soap

(b) For the base of glycerol-gelatin

Arachis oil or liquid paraffin are used as lubricants.

The preparation process:-

When making suppositories using the fusion method, always add the weight of an additional 2 suppositories to account for material loss during transfer. Take the appropriate amount of medicine and base for 10 suppositories, for instance, if you wish to produce 8 suppositories. Following the instructions above, thoroughly clean and lube the mould. Keepmould is placed upside-down on an ice bath to drain the mould cavity of any extra lubricants. Melt the foundation for the suppository in a porcelain dish over water, then whisk in the medicine. Place excess of this substance in the mould cavity before setting the mould in an ice bath. Open the mould when the extra mount has solidified. Remove the suppository, wrap it in waxed paper or tin foil, and place it in the appropriate container.

Automated moulding apparatus:-

On an automatic rotational moulding machine, several moulding activities like pouring, cooling, and removal are carried out. Both the cleaning of the mould and the ejection of hardened suppositories are totally automated. A rotating machine can produce between 3500 and 6000 suppositories each hour in large-scale production.

Problems associated with preparation of suppositories

- Water in suppositories
- Hygroscopicity
- Incompatibilities
- Viscosity
- Density
- Volume contraction
- Brittleness
- Lubricant or mould release agent
- Weight and volume control
- Rancidity
- Some marketed formulation of suppositories

1. Dulcolax Suppositories (Bisacodyl 10 mg).

   Use: Constipation that necessitates the use of a stimulant laxative, whether it be recent or persistent.

2. Tyridol Suppositories (Tramadol hydrochloride 100 mg).

Use: Anti-inflammatory

3. Galipar 125 (Children), Galipar 500 (Adult) Suppositories (Acetaminophen 125 mg for children and 500 mg for adult).

   Use: Antipyretic.

4. Hallens Adult/Child Suppositories (Glycerin 75% w/w).

   Use Laxative.

5. Proctosedyl® Suppositories (Hydrocortisone 5 mg and cinchocaine 5 mg).

   Use. To treat hemorrhoids and itching/swelling in the rectum and anus

Displacement Value:-

Although the suppository is prepared by weight, a suppository mould is filled by volume. Due to the differing densities of the base and medication, the weight of a suppository created from a particular mould can change when a pharmaceutical is present.

The amount of medication needed to move one component of the base is represented by the displacement value.

Calculation of Value Displacement:

The displacement value of a specific drug can be determined using the following method if it is unknown:-

1.10 suppositories should be prepared and weighed using just the base. Let these weigh what they weigh 'A' gramme

2. Make and weigh ten suppositories with a given amount of a (medicated suppository). These should weigh "B" grammes.

3. Determine how much base is in the prescription suppositories. Let the weight-loss be "C"gram.

4 Determine how much medication is in each suppository. Let the dosage be in"D" gram.

5.As a result, (A-C) will represent the base's weight that the medication has moveD

6.The medication's displacement value for a specific base will be ;

Value of displacement = D/ (A-C)

Examples:-

(1)Calculate actual weight of cocoa butter required to prepare 10 suppositories, each containing 0.2 g of drug of displacement value 4.

Solution: Since 1 g weight suppository mould is used Total weight of cocoa butter alone required for preparation of 10 suppositories :

1 × 10 =10 g

As each suppository should contain 0.2 g of drug, hence total weight of drug required to prepare 10 suppositories is

0.2×10=2g

According to displacement value, 8 g of drug will displace 1 g of cocoa butter therefore 2 g of drug will displace 2×1/4 = 0.5 g of cocoa butter

Hence, actual quantity of cocoa butter required to prepare 15 suppositories will be:

10 – 0.5 = 9.5g

Therefore,

Total weight of 10 suppositories will;

9.5 (cocoa butter) + 2 g (drug) = 16.75 g i.e.

It shows that even if suppositories are made in a 1 g mould, their volume remains the same but their weight is larger than 1 g.

(2)Find the medication's displacement value in a cocoa butter suppository that contains 40% of the drug and was made in a 1 g mould. 10 suppositories weigh 14.72 g.

Weight of 10 suppositories made in a 1 g mould and only containing cocoa butter.

1x 10 = 10 g

Given is the weight of 10 suppositories carrying 40% of the medication. = 14.72 g

The amount of cocoa butter in a medicated suppository (which contains 60% of the drug)

14.72 g = 100%

X g = 60 %

X= 14.72 ×60/100 = 8.83 g

Amount of drug present in medicated suppository (containing 40 % of drug):

14.72 g = 100%

X g = 40 %

X= 14.72 × 40/100 = 5.89 g

Amount of cocoa butter displaced by 6.184g of drug

= 10 – 8.83 = 1.17 g

Therefore, displacement value :

Displacement value = 5.89 / 1.17 = 5.03

Displacement value of few drugs with reference to cocoa butter as a suppository bases:-

Name of drug	Displacement value	Name of drug	Displacement value
Alum	2.0	Ichthammol	1.0
Aminophyline	1.5	Iodoform	4.0
Aspirin	1.1	Boric Acid	1.5
Bismuth subgallate	3.0	Phenobarbitone	1.0
Hydrocortisone acetate	1.5	Resorcinol	1.0
Castor oil	1.0	Tannic Acid	1.0
Chloral hydrate	1.5	Zinc Oxide	5.0
Cocaine Hydrochloride	1.5	Zinc Sulphate	2.0

EVALUATION OF SUPPOSITORIES :-

Prepared suppositories are evaluated for following quality control test;

1.Visual inspection: It's important to check the suppository for any signs of drug migration, fat blossoming, exudation, or fissuring pitting. Suppositories are examined both whole and after being split longitudinally.

In the suppositories' test shape of suppositories, homogeneity of colours and surface condition are visually inspection is done for things like brilliance, dullness, mottling, cracks, dark areas in the axial cavities, bursts, air bubbles, holes, etc.

2.Odor: When comparable suppositories are used, confirming the odour might help avoid confusion being handled. Additionally, a change in odour could be a sign of deterioration.

process.

3.Weight variation test: Weigh each of the 20 suppositories separately to ascertain

typical weight Compared to the average weight, compare the individual weights. Except for two that may differ by no more than 10%, no suppository should deviate from average weight by more than 5%. Weight fluctuation in suppositories may be caused by improper scraping, air entrapment, or mould voids that are either under- or over-filled.

4.Identifying the melting point: Several methods, such as the open capillary tube, the U-tube, and the drop point procedures, are used to research melting behaviour. Utilizing a U-shaped capillary tube to evaluate the melting point of suppositories that include soluble active principles gives manufacturers precise information for excipient management and manufacturing consistency. High powder content in suppositories makes it impossible for the fat to slide inside the capillary tube to provide the end-point determination, making them unsuitable for this approach.

5.A small-diameter wire inserted into the mould containing the suppository melt just before the form solidifies can also be used to determine the melting point. When the suppository slides off the wire while being held by the wire and the form is submerged in water, it has reached its melting point. This is accomplished by gradually raising the liquid's temperature (by roughly 1°C every 2–3 minutes).

6.Melting range test: This test is used to evaluate the suppository's physical and absorption qualities. The macro melting range test is another name for this test. The amount of time needed for the complete suppository to melt at a constant temperature, such as 37°C. USP tablet disintegration test equipment is employed for this test. The time it takes for the complete test suppository to melt or scatter in the surrounding water is timed while it is fully submerged in the continuous water bath.

7.Liquification or softening time test: Liquefaction testing reveals how a suppository behaves when exposed to a temperature of up to 37°C. Krowczynski's method is used to calculate the suppository's liquefaction or softening time, which estimates the amount of time needed for a suppository to liquefy at pressures comparable to those encountered in the rectum (about 30 g) when water is present at 37°C. Liquefaction generally shouldn't take more than 30 minutes.

The mechanical strength/crushing test: It determines the amount of force required to break a suppository and reveals whether it is elastic or brittle. This test makes use of the Erweka methodology. According to the Erweka technique, the mechanical strength shouldn't be less than 1.8 to 2 kg. The test's goal is to confirm that the suppository can be transferred and given to the patient in a normal setting.

8.Deformation Time: This is the amount of time that a suppository can maintain its original shape while being subjected to a certain amount of pressure. By placing a known weight on a suppository inside a known pH medium at a specified temperature of no higher than 37°C, this can be ascertained. The suppository's deformation time is the length of time it takes to lose its shape.

9.Content homogeneity. By checking suppositories at random for drug content uniformity in accordance with guidelines provided in the relevant pharmacopoeia, the dosage to dose variance can be reduced. Pharmaceutical Codex 1993 mandates that preparations of suppositories with active ingredients less than 2g or 2% of the total masses must pass the test for content homogeneity. Using an appropriate assay method, the active component content of each of the suppositories that were chosen at random for this test should be identified.

For suppositories, acceptance value calculations are not necessary. Unless otherwise specified in the Procedure for content uniformity, assay 10 units separately as instructed in the Assay in the particular monograph. The following restrictions on content consistency are stated in the USP 30 Criteria for suppositories.

Limit A: (If the sum of the limits listed in the individual monograph's definition of potency is 100.0% or less). As determined by the Content Uniformity approach, the amount of the drug substance in each of the 10 dosage units falls between 85% and 115% of the label claim, and the relative standard deviation is less than or equal to 69%, unless differently stated in the particular monograph. twenty more units for testing if no units fall outside of the range of 75% to 125% of the label claim, if the relative standard deviation is greater than 6.0%, if both requirements are met, or if 1 unit deviates from the label claim's range of 85% to 115%..

The standards are satisfied if no more than one of the 30 dosage units deviates from the label claim by more than 85% to 115%, no unit deviates from the label claim by more than 75% to 125%, and the 30 dosage units' relative standard deviation does not go over 7.8%.

Limit B: (If the mean of the thresholds listed in the potency specification in the specific monograph is higher than 100.0 percent). If the average value of the dose units examined is 100.0 percent or less, the requirements are the same as in Limit A. With the exception that "label claim" is changed to "label claim multiplied by the average of the limitations provided in the potency definition in the monograph divided by 100," the requirements are the same as those under Limit A. if the average of the dose units tested exceeds or is equivalent to the average of the limitations listed in the specific monograph's definition of potency.

With the exception that "label claim" is substituted by "label claim multiplied by the average value of the dosage units tested (expressed as a percent of label claim) divided by 100," the requirements are the same as those in Limit A. This is true if the dosage units' average value falls within the range of the limitations listed in the potency definition in the particular monograph, which is between 100 percent and the average of those limits.

10.Dissolution Test : One of the most crucial quality control tools for in-vitro testing is the dissolution study. According to FDA regulations, suppository dissolving testing must also check for hardening and polymorphic transitions of the active components and suppository bases. Suppositories are tested for suppository disintegration using the Basket, Paddle, and Beaker procedures. Diffusion, dialysis, and continuous flow methods are available. However, Unlike tablets and capsule dosage forms, there aren't enough dissolving testing methods or validations for suppositories. This can be due to the water immiscibility of some suppository delivery systems.

After careful deliberation, the US FDA came to the conclusion that the basket, paddle, or flow-through cell procedures can be used to evaluate hydrophilic suppositories that release the medicine by dissolving in the rectal secretions. On the other hand, lipophilic suppositories, which melt in the rectal cavity and are significantly impacted by rectal temperature, release the drug after doing so. It follows that modified flow-through cells with particular dual-chamber suppository cells, a paddle method with a wired screen and a sinker, and a modified basket method are all recommended equipment for lipophilic suppositories.

11.Studies on Product Stability: According to the USP, product stability refers to the degree to which a product maintains its properties during the course of storage and usage, as long as those conditions are met (i.e. shelf life). In a stability research, suppositories are placed in containers at the appropriate temperatures and relative humidity levels, and evaluations must be made of their shape, colour, assay, degradation products, particle size, softening range, dissolving (at 37°C), and microbiological limitations.

QUESTIONS

Short Answer Questions

1. What are suppositories?
2. What do understand by term bougies?
3. What is the importance of calibration of mould?
4. What are the various lubricants used to lubricate the mould?
5. What is displacement value?
6. What are pessaries?

Long Answer Questions

1.What are the ideal properties of suppository bases?
2. Define suppositories and its various types.
3.Discuss various methods of preparing suppositories.
4. What are the advantages and disadvantages of theobroma oil as suppository base?
5.What are the evaluation methods of suppositories?
6.Write in brief about displacement value?
7.How will you find displacement value of the medicament?
8.Explain different methods for preparation of suppository.
9.Write a note on:
(i)Calibration of suppository mould
(ii) Cocoa butter as a suppository base
(iii)Recent development in suppositories
(iv) Packaging of suppositories

CHAPTER XII

PHARMACEUTICAL INCOMPATIBILITIES

A pharmaceutical incompatibility may be defined as the result when medications that are inherently antagonistic are prescribed or mixed, an unwanted product is produced that may compromise the preparation's safety purpose or appearance. OR When two or more antagonistic substances are combined, compatibility results, and an unwanted product is created that may impact the safety, effectiveness, and appearance of the pharmaceutical preparation. Compounding and dispensing are just two instances of when incompatibility might happen. It can also happen at any point during drug formulation, production, packaging, or administration.

Types of Incompatibilities:-

1. Physical incompatibility
2. Chemical incompatibility
3. Therapeutic incompatibility

(A) Physical incompatibility

A physical change occurs when two or more substances are combined, resulting in the formation of an undesirable product. Physical incompatibility is primarily caused by solid materials' insolubility, immiscibility, precipitation, or liquefaction. These modifications that result from physical Using pharmaceutical expertise to create a suitable preparation, these modifications can be quickly addressed because they are frequently observed.are typically obvious, can be easily fixed, look nice, and can be made with enough therapeutic effect with pharmacological skill.Any one or more of the following techniques can be used to address the physical incompatibilities uniform dosage:

Any one or more of the following techniques can be used to address the physical incompatibilities uniform dosage: -

1. Immiscibility observation
2. Combined insolubility
3. Liquefaction

a. Immiscibility

a. Oils and water cannot mix, thus when water and oily medications are combined, the result is a product with two distinct layers. Solution: Emulsification or solubilization can solve this issue.
b. When using concentrated hydroalcoholic solutions of volatile oils, like spirits and concentrated waters, are used as adjuncts (like flavoring agents) in preparations of aqueous media, specific procedures must be followed.Oils form distinct layers in large molecules or globules.Solution:Either the vehicle or the hydroalcoholic solution should be added.

while being constantly stirred, or it should be gradually diluted with the vehicle before being combined with the other ingredients. This will prevent the production of big globules.

c.When the prescription contains a significant amount of potassium citrate, the spirit of ethyl nitrite separates and floats as a layer.

d. The vehicle is a saturated aqueous solution of a volatile oil in which high concentrations of electrolytes, such as salts, are added.For instance, the oil separates and accumulates into an unsightly surface layer.

4 Potassium Citrate Mixture B.P.C. When lemon spirit, which is used as a flavoring, is added, the solution salts out because of the high concentration of soluble salt and the change in solvent. This makes the solution salty (potassium citrate).As an emulsifier, quillaia tincture is added to prevent this oil from separating from the surface layer..

b. Insolubility

a. Some insoluble powders, including sulphru and some antibiotics and corticosteroids (hydrocortisone acetate) are challenging to moisten with water.

Remedy -Wetting agents like saponins for sulphur containing lotions and polysorbate in parental suspensions of corticosteroids . b.The precipitation of acacia by the alcohol gives the mixture of mucilage of acacia and alcohol the appearance of being unpleasant. Acacia can be omitted from the preparation to prevent this conflict and still produce a good product. c. The suspension created in liquid medicines with diffusible particles settles quickly, making it impossible to pour out consistent doses. In these situations, a thickening agent is used to boost viscosity and slow down particle settling.

d. The suspension created in liquid medicines containing indiffusible materials settles quickly, making it impossible to pour out consistent doses.

For instance, chalk, aromatic chalk powder, succinyl sulfathiazole and sulphadimidine (mixed), calamine and zinc oxide (in lotion), and chalk. Remedy for this is to add thickening agents such as gum acacia, gum tragacanth, methylcellulose etc. to increase the viscosity and reduce the rate of settling of particles.

c. Liquefaction

When various distinct low melting point particles are powdered together, the mixture's melting point drops to below room temperature, resulting in a liquid or soft mass.Consequently, a eutectic mixture emerges.Any two of the following are examples of this kind of conduct:chloral hydrate, camphor, phenazone, thymol, sodium salicylate, and menthol.

(1) For instance, when two parts of salol and one part of menthol are combined, a syrupy liquid results, whereas when one part of salol and one part of menthol are combined, a moist powder results. But a dry mixture is made up of one component salol and two parts menthol.

i. When rubbed together, substances such as acetanilid, antipyrine, betanaphthol, resorcinol, thymol, etc. may also liquefy.
ii. Menthol and thymol are triturated in a mortar to create the liquid mixture if they must be administered as a powder. A sufficient amount of adsorbent powder, such as light kaolin or light magnesium carbonate, is added to the liquid during trituration to produce a free-flowing end product. If the final bulk volume of powder is very little, another approach can be applied. Thymol and menthol are are each independently triturated with a little quantity

of adsorbent powder. The two powders are then easily mixed, and the resulting powder is put into capsules .The absorbent granules cover the particle to keep the medications from coming into contact with one another and to absorb any liquid that might be created during trituration.

d. Wrong form of the ingredients prescribed:- Alkaloidal salts may need to be dissoved in the liquid petroleum but when the alkaloid is used instead, the alkaloidal salt dissolves completely. While alkaloidal salts are insoluble in liquid petrolatum, free alkaloids are soluble in it.
e. Gelatinization: The addition of ferric salts causes the acacia solution to

gelatinize. Phenol is also added to collodion to gelatinize it. Remedies for physical incompatibilities:-

1. Omission of an unimportant ingredient of little therapeutic value.
2. Addition of an inert ingredient to correct the difficulty.

3.alteration in the solvents used (water being replaced with alcohol or glycerin, or the other way around)

4.altering the order in which the ingredients are mixed.

5.distributing the components one at a time.

6.modifying the majority of the three preparation.7.utilizing a distinct formulation of the same ingredient.8.Stiffening agents being added,

7.Addition of an ingredient which promotes solubility.

(B) Chemical Incompatibility

When two substances are chemically incompatible, a new, unfavourable product is created as a result of the chemical reaction. Chemical reactions between the constituents cause incompatibility, and the resultant product may

be inactive or dangerous. These kinds of incompatibilities can be hard to fix, and in some cases, it may be necessary to get rid of or replace one of the reacting substances, put them in separate containers, make them non-reactive, or pack and store them in the right containers. In such cases, a doctor should be informed. To avoid the production of hazardous products, measures should be taken when dispensing such preparations. Oxidation-reduction, acid-base hydrolysis, or combination reactions are the causes of chemical incompatibilities. Precipitation, effervescence, breakdown, and colour changes result from these processes or by detonation. Two categories of chemical incompatibility exist:

1. Tolerable: -When mixing solutions in diluted form or in different order than usual, the chemical interaction is reduced to a minimum.
2. Modified:- In modified incompatibilities, a prescription's reactive chemicals are added to or substituted with another substance to prevent a chemical interaction another with equivalent therapeutic benefit The incompatibility could be due to intentional: When a doctor purposefully prescribes the medications that are not compatible with one another; ii. Unintentional: -When the physician gives the drugs without realising that they are incompatible prescription medications.

1) Incompatibility with Alkaloids

Examples:

a)Alkaloids are weak bases, thus they go well with alkaline compounds. While
alkaloidal salts are soluble in water, they are nearly insoluble. The free

12 alkaloid may precipitate when these salts are added to alkaline solutions like sodium bicarbonate, strong ammonium acetate solution, aromatic ammonia spirit, solution of ammonia, and ammonium bicarbonate.Alkaloidal salts with salicylates: Quinine compounds react with salicylates to generate indiffusible quinine salicylate precipitates.

2. Incompatibilities with soluble salicylates

Ferric salt interacts with sodium salicylate to release insoluble precipitates of ferric salicylate.

3. Chemical incompatibilities that lead to carbon dioxide gas evolution .In a mixture, carbonates and bicarbonates react when they come into touch with an acid or an acidic substance, causing carbon dioxide gas to be released. If the reaction is not allowed to finish before the mixture is put into a dispensing bottle and corked, there is a danger that the bottle will explode. Before releasing the combination, the reaction must be finished to prevent explosion. The

materials were combined in an open jar to hasten the reaction, and it was let to run its course until the effervescence subsided.

(b) Gas evolution:- Combining an acid with carbonate or bicarbonate

(should To prevent explosions, compounds are made in open containers. (c) Color alterations: Alterations in colour brought on by a chemical reaction or the creation of a new substance.

d. Explosion production:- An explosion happens when a potent oxidising agent is triturated with reducing agents or organic materials. Explosions are caused by the abrupt evolution of gases, hence extreme caution must be used when handling any compounds that could result in such a gaseous evolution after being triturated.
e. Cementation of materials:- In some circumstances, all or a portion of a prescription's ingredients may solidify into a mass with a hardness akin to cement. separation of an impermeable liquid when an organic chemical, such as the, is broken down by a specific reagent, degraded by a specific reagent, such as when an alkali transforms chloral into chloroform.
f. The impact of pH: -Modern medications are frequently salts of weak acids and bases. While free bases are essentially insoluble in water, these salts are typically soluble. As a result, when a weak acid salt solution is acidified, the free weak acid may precipitate out. Similar to this, the free weak base may precipitate out of an alkaline solution of a weak base salt. The solubility of the unionised acid or base, the pH of the solution, or the dissociation constant (K) of the acid or base determine whether or not precipitation occurs.
g. Alkaloidal salts with double breakdown, such as emetine hydrochloride Alkaloids precipitate as insoluble iodide salts after reacting with soluble potassium iodide. Since emetine-HI is less soluble, it may precipitate. For instance, certain cough medicines containing alkaloid employ potassium iodide as an expectorant. Precipitation does not happen if the alkaloid content is very low. Alkaloidal salts and tannins are incompatible, which is another illustration of this type. Alkaloidal tannates are precipitated when alkaloidal salts and tannins interact. The benefit of this reaction is that the alkaloids can be precipitated in cases of alkaloidal poisoning using strong tea or a tannic acid solution. Precipitate must be suspended using tragacanth mucilage as a cure.

Remedies for Chemical compatibility :-

1. As directed in the following prescription, add glycerin, syrup, or honey to the incompatible ingredients before mixing to prevent precipitation.
2. During the preparation of the codeine sulphate solution, a slight turbidity develops as a result of the formation of codeine tannate as well as the separation of the resinous matter from the aromatic syrup. However A clear solution is produced when the three codeine salts are triturated in a vehicle that is equal parts glycerin and fragrant eriodyctiol syrup.
3. A violent reaction occurs when iodine is added directly to oil of turpentine. The mixture could possibly catch fire due to the amount of heat produced. However, the reaction will be greatly reduced even though some heat may emerge when the iodine is first diluted in alcohol before being gradually added to the turpentine oil .Mixing should ideally take place in an open container.
4. A thick, white precipitate of quinine acetate is produced when quinine sulphate is dissolved in sulfuric acid and combined with a solution of sodium acetate. The sodium acetate is partially transformed into acetic acid and sodium sulphate. However, if the acid is left out, quinine sulphate is formed in a fine solution. There is some conversion of the sodium acetate into sodium sulfate and 3 acetic acid.On the other hand, if the acid is not used, a fine suspension of quinine sulfate is produced. This should be labeled "shake well" because it should be shaken

well.

5. When first formulated, zinc sulphate The solution is clear, but eventually there might be a precipitation of the barely soluble basic zinc borate, which is not good for the eyes. Boric acid can be used in place of sodium borate to avoid precipitation.

(C) Therapeutic Incompatibility

A sort of pharmacological incompatibility called a therapeutic incompatibility, also known as a physiological incompatibility, occurs when the recommended medications have an unfavourable in vivo effect and also Usually this incompatibility arises while one or greater tablets produces reaction or depth distinctive from that meant withinside the patients. It can be because of following beneath stated reasons:

There are two different sorts of therapeutic incompatibility mechanisms involved:

1. Pharmacokinetics: This mechanism relates to how one drug affects how another drug is absorbed, distributed, metabolised, and excreted.
2. Pharmacodynamics: This mechanism relates to the pharmacological effects of the drugs that interact with each other, including synergism, antagonistic effects, altered cellular transport, and effects on the receptor site. Therapeutic Incompatibility Causes:

I. Interactions with Pharmacokinetics

1. Modified GIT absorption: This type involves changes to the bacterial flora, pH, and formation of chelates for drugs altered GIT motility and mucosal injury brought on by complexes and drugs is a factor in drug incompatibility.

a. Changed pH: Drugs in their non-ionized form are more lipid soluble and more easily absorbed from the gastrointestinal tract than their ionised counterparts and drugs such as ketoconazole tablets. In such situations, these drugs should be administered by the difference of at least duration of 2h interval in the time of administration .
b. Complexation or chelation: Tetracycline interacts with calcium (present in milk) or iron (Hematinic preparations) to form chelates that are not absorbed through intestinal tract. Another example is antacids such as aluminum or magnesium hydroxide interacts with ciprofloxacin reducing its absorption by 85% due to chelate formation. Thus care must be taken to avoid administration of such substances together.
c. Drug-induced mucosal damage: Anti-neoplastic agents such as Cyclophos phamide, vincristine and procarbazine inhibit absorption of digoxin.
d. Altered motility: An antiemetic drug metoclopramide increases stomach emptying time. This drug increases absorption of cyclosporine which may be toxic.

2. Displaced protein binding

The drug's affinity for plasma protein determines how well it binds to proteins. Most likely bound drugs can take the place of other drugs.By being replaced by another drug with a higher affinity, the free drug is increased in quantity .Phenytoin, for instance, is highly bound to warfarin, tolbutamide, and plasma protein. Phenylbutazone, sulfonamides, and aspirin displaces phenytoin which remains as free form and is highly absorbed thus may exert toxic effects.

3. Altered metabolism

There are examples of drugs that effect metabolism of the other drugs changing its effectiveness. Although liver is the major site of drug metabolism, other organs WBC, skin, lung, and GIT can also contribute for the same. Enzyme induction: A drug may induce the enzyme that is responsible metabolism of another drug or as itself too .

(b) for example: Carbamazepine, an antiepileptic, increases its own metabolism. Phenytoin, on the other hand, increases hepatic metabolism, lowering theophylline's level and activity. The maximum effect of enzyme induction takes about three weeks because it involves protein synthesis.Inhibition of enzymes:Enzyme inhibition slows down the metabolism of drugs by a different enzyme raises the concentration of the target medication, increasing its toxicity. Competition at binding sites may be the cause of the enzyme's inhibition, which accounts for its rapid commencement of activity. For instance, when verapamil, an inhibitor, is supplied along with carbamazepine, an enzyme inducer, the inhibitor's impact, which is more pronounced, alters the concentration of carbamazepine and, eventually, its effect. Erythromycin's ability to block the metabolism of astemazole and terfenadine is another illustration of this sort. A rise in the potentially fatal cardiotoxicity is caused by an increase in the serum levels of antihistaminic drugs. Diazepam's oxidative metabolism is inhibited by omeprazole.

(b) First-pass metabolism: Giving a medicine orally increases the likelihood that it will be metabolized in the liver and GIT causing some of the drug dose to be lost, which lessens the drug's effectiveness. When using a medicine that either induces or inhibits enzymes, this effect is more pronounced. For instance, verapamil's hepatic metabolism is induced by rifampin, which lowers the serum level of verapamil.

4. Modified renal function

a. Proximal renal tubules experience inhibition of renal tubular secretion. To get through the proximal tubules, the medication joins forces with a certain protein. Drug excretion is decreased, its concentration is raised, and consequently its toxicity when a substance has a competitive reactivity to the protein (which is in charge of the active transport of another substance). Probenecid, for instance, reduces methotrexate's tubular secretion.
b. Changes in urine flow and pH: Drugs are excreted and reabsorbed.

Pharmacodynamic Interactions:-

It means alteration of the drug without change in its serum concerntrations.

1. Over doses
2. Under doses
3. Contraindicated tablets
4. Drug interactions

a) Over Doses

Overuse of a single dose:Depending on the person's health, a single dose can sometimes also be an overdose; for instance, a daily dose (assuming a body weight of 70 kg as the standard for an adult male) can be an overdose for a person who is underweight.

a. A capsule with 360 mg of phenobarbital and 6 mg of atropine sulphate to be taken three times a day before meals.This capsule contains 12 times the normal dose of both phenobarbital and atropine sulphate 1.The doctor wants to give 12 capsules, but maybe they did it wrong or the prescription was wrong.Atropine sulphate 6 mg and phenobarbital 360 mg to be dispensed in total 12 capsules with the label stating "One capsule to be taken three times a day before meals" should therefore be reviewed by the pharmacist prior to dispensing.

b. a 500 mg capsule containing 500 mg of iron, ammonium citrate, and strychnine sulphate.Three times per day, one capsule should be taken after meals.The normal dose of strychnine hydrochloride is ten times higher than this one.The physician should be consulted by the one pharmacist before a dose adjustment can be made.Therefore, the prescription must be amended to include 500 mg of iron and 500 mg of ammonium citrate and strychnine sulphate.One capsule, three times a day, one after each meal.
c. Excessive dosage every day:The drug's daily dose has been exceeded in this instance.For instance, a capsule containing 500 mg of ammonium 1 chloride and 15 mg of codeine phosphate.For cough, take two capsules every hour.Instead of taking the prescribed dose every hour, the U.S.P. suggests taking it every four hours.As a result, you should talk to your doctor.
d. Effect of addition:When two or more drugs with the same effect combine, the combined effect is the sum of their individual effects at different doses.The client may benefit or suffer from this additive effect.Similar pharmacological activity can be found in some drugs.The physician's advice is required in this situation.For instance, a 100 mL mixture of amphetamine sulphate 20 mg and ephedrine sulphate 50 mg in syrup base with a 25 mL dose every four hoursIn this particular instance, both medications, which are sympathetic stimulants, are prescribed in full dosage.The formulation will have the effect of an additive overdose.As a result, each drug's dosage should be decreased.
e. Effect of synergy:When two or more drugs with or without the same effect are given together to produce a combined effect that is greater than the sum of the active components of each drug, this is called a synergistic effect.When combined with verapamil, propranolol has a synergistic effect.
f. Effect of potential:The term "potentiating effect" refers to a specific kind of synergistic effect that occurs when two drugs interact, but only one of them has an effect that is made stronger by the presence of the other.Diuretics, for instance, lower the potassium concentration in the blood and, as a result, enhance digoxin's effects and increase the risk of glycoside toxicity.
g. negative effects:Reactions that have the opposite effect of synergy and produce a combined effect that is less than that of either active component on its own are known as antagonistic effects.Protamine, for instance, is used to counteract the effects of anticoagulants.

Example- Prescription Atropine sulfate, 6 mg Phenobarbital, 360 mg CapsulesLabel:One capsule should be taken three times per afternoon, just before meals.1 Method: Phenobarbital and atropine sulphate are both prescribed at 12 times the usual dose in this prescription.The doctor intended to prescribe 12 capsules, but he may have written the prescription incorrectly or insufficiently.As a result, the pharmacist ought to seek the advice of the doctor once more before dispensing the medication.

Proper prescription: a prescription for phenobarbital 360 mg in capsule form.Provide 12 capsules Label:Take one capsule daily. 3 instances an afternoon earlier than meals.

Example

RX

Iron, strychnine sulfate, and ammonium citrate, 500 milligrams Each capsule should contain 12 pills.

Label:One capsule should be taken three times per afternoon, immediately after meals.

Comment:Strychnine hydrochloride overdose at ten times the normal levelThe doctor should give the pharmacist permission to change one of the doses, so they should.

Prescription modification:Ammonium citrate -500 mg and strychnine sulfate - 2 mg Make capsules.Provide 12 capsules.1 Label:One capsule should be taken three times per afternoon, immediately after meals.Excessive dosage daily:In this instance, the drug's daily dose is exceeded.Ephedrine sulfate 50 mg syrup q.s. - 100 ml Mix the ingredients together.Label:Take 25 ml every four hours.1 Method:The two medications work together to enhance one another.Overdose will have an effect on the system.As a result, each drug's dosage needs to be decreased.

2.Under dose

In this type of incompatibility, the effect of one drug is diminished or counteracted by the presence of another drug.This can be demonstrated by combining the first of the following drugs.1.stimulants like caffeine, nuxvomica, and others.with a variety of sedatives, including paraldehyde and barbiturates.1

2.Castor oil, liquid paraffin, and numerous other purgatives with antidiarrheal properties like bismuth carbonates are examples.3.Alkalizers like sodium bicarbonate, magnesium carborate, and Rx Aspirin -300 mg Probenecid -500 mg can be used as acidifiers.Label:For gout, take one capsule each afternoon.In the event of a gout attack, aspirin is taken to reduce pain and swelling.While salicylates (aspirin) prevent probenecid from moving through the kidney lumen, probenecid prevents the active reabsorption of uric acid.As a result, the medications are incompatible with one another, rendering their combination therapeutically ineffective.

3. Contraindicated Drug:- some drugs should be avoided in some conditions. For Example :-

Patients with peptic ulcers should not take corticosteroids.ii.

Vasoconstrictors shouldn't be used on people who have high blood pressure.

Certain medications are contraindicated.To make capsules, add 0.25 g of sulphadiazine, 0.25 g of sulphamerazine, and 0.50 g of ammonium chloride. For cough, take six capsules every hour.

Comment: Ammonium chloride, which is in this prescription, can make the urine more acidic and put sulphonamide crystals in the kidney.

4. Drug Interactions

The impact of 1 drug is altered with the aid of using the earlier or simultaneous management of any other drug. The drug interactions can commonly be corrected with the aid of using the right adjustment of dosage if the suspected interaction is detected.

Example:9Acetophenetidin -150 milligrams Acetyl salicylic acid -200 milligrams Caffeine -30 milligrams Send ten capsules Acetophenetidin depresses the central nervous system, which is a negative side effect.Caffeine is a CNS stimulant that counteracts the acetophenetidin side effect.

The incompatibility is made up on purpose.

Example:

Rx Tetracycline hydrochloride -250 milligrams Make 10 capsules and distribute them.

Label:

Consume one capsule once every six hours.

Comments: Because milk's calcium inactivates the tetracycline, taking the capsule with milk may not provide any therapeutic benefit.The patient should be advised by the pharmacist to take the pill with water, not milk, as a remedy. The patient shouldn't use calcium salts-containing antacids.

CHAPTER XIII

SEMISOLID DOSAGE FORMS

OBJECTIVES

Semisolid dosage forms are pharmaceutical formulations that often come in the type of creams, gels, ointments, or pastes and include one or more active agents that have been uniformly dissolved or dispersed in a suitable base and any relevant excipients. These are some of the chapter's goals :

- To learn fundamental concepts, as well as the benefits and drawbacks of semisolids.
- Recognize the dosage form categorization, the mechanism impacting medication skin penetration, and the route of drug administration.
- To gain a comprehensive understanding of the different bases and excipients used, as well as formulation concerns for developing semisolid products.
- To comprehend manufacturing process and the varied physical characteristics of semisolids.

INTRODUCTION

Semisolids are topical dose formulations with medical, protective, or cosmetic use. They can be used topically, on the eye's surface, or nasally, vaginally, or rectally. Ointments, pastes, creams, plasters, gels are the semisolid formulations. They include any relevant excipients, such as emulsifiers, thickeners, antibacterial agents, antioxidants, stabilizing agents, etc., as well as one or more active ingredients that have been dissolved or uniformly dispersed in a suitable base.

Gels, creams, and ointments are semisolid dose forms designed for topical use. Most of these formulations are meant to enhance the therapeutic effects of the drugs they contain. Due to its physical effects, unmedicated ones are utilised as a lubricant or protector. Both local and systemic effects can be achieved using topical medicines. If the patient is pregnant or breastfeeding, systemic medicine absorption should always be taken into account before using topical treatments since medications can enter the fetal blood supply and be passed to the fetus through breast milk. Both local effects and systemic absorption are possible with topical operations. Regarding dermatologic surgeries, the following differentiation is crucial. Topical dermatological product is made to treat dermal disorders with the skin as the target organ by delivering medication directly into the skin. With the skin not being the target organ, a transdermal product is made to carry medications via the skin to the general circulation for systemic effects.

IDEAL PROPERTY OF SEMISOLID DOSAGE FORM

IDEAL PROPERTY OF SEMISOLID DOSAGE FORM			
Physical properties	**Physiological properties**	**Application properties**	**Storage properties**
Smooth texture	Non-irritating	Effortlessly applicable	Not exceed 25 ° degrees
Elegant in appearance	Do not alter membrane / skin functioning	High aqueous washing ability	Stored in a well closed vessel
Non-greasy and non-staining	Miscible with skin secretion		Not be allowed to freeze
Non-hygroscopic	Low sensitization index		

Fig:1.1 Ideal Property of Semisolid Dosage Form

Advantages :

1. It is externally applied.

1. The affected area is subject to local and site-specific effects of the medication.

3. It is a more stable dose form than liquid.

4. Side effects may be less likely.

5. Easy to provide orally for a patient who is unconscious.

6. Hepatic and intestinal first pass metabolism is avoided.

7. Appropriate for bitter medications.

Disadvantages :

1. There is less dose precision with this kind of dosing form.

2. For certain patients, it might irritate or trigger an allergy.

3. It might leave stains.

4. Contamination can result from applying a medication with your finger.

5. As they are bulky, difficult to handle.

6. Physico-chemical stability is higher for solid dose forms than semisolid dosage forms.

CLASSIFICATION OF SEMISOLID DOSAGE FORMS

Semisolid formulations include ointments, pastes, creams, gels, plasters and etc .

1. **Ointments :**

The base is the ingredient or element of an ointment or other semisolid preparation that acts as the medication's carrier or vehicle. The preference of a suitable base for an ointment or cream formulation is influenced by the desired activity (for example, topical or percutaneous absorption), ease of manufacture, compatibility with other ingredients, pourability and spreadability of the formulation, physicochemical and microbial stability of the product, duration of contact, likelihood of hypersensitivity reactions, and ease of washing from the application site. Moreover, bases used in ophthalmic preparations should not irritate skin and soften at body temperatures.

Following factors affect ointment base selection.

- Desired rate of drug ingredient release from ointment base.
- Topical or transcutaneous medication absorption volume and rate.
- Desirability of blocking skin moisture.
- Drug stability in the ointment base.
- Drug's impact on the base's consistency.
- On washing base should easily get removes.

Based on their composition and physical features, ointment bases are categorised. Ointment bases are categorised as follows by the United States Pharmacopeia :

i. Oleaginous bases (Hydrocarbon bases)
ii. Absorption bases
iii. Water soluble bases
iv. Water-miscible bases

i. Oleaginous bases :

Oleaginous bases are also known as Hydrocarbon bases. This are non-aqueous formulations that provide long-lasting emollient and protecting effects on the skin. Aqueous phases are challenging to integrate into hydrocarbon bases. However, using liquid petrolatum, powders can be integrated into these bases. Because of the greasy nature, hydrocarbon bases are challenging to remove from the skin. The following elements are present in hydrocarbon bases: Hard paraffin , soft paraffin, liquid paraffin , white/yellow soft paraffin, mineral oil, and microcrystalline wax.

The advantages of hydrocarbon bases:

- Emollients prevent moisture loss from the application site by creating an occlusive film that prevents moisture loss and maintains the skin soft.
- They can tolerate heat sterilisation, thus it can be used to make sterile ophthalmic ointments.
- They are very nearly inert. They mostly consist of saturated hydrocarbons, thus there are fewer incompatibilities and rancidity tendencies.
- Since they are sticky, the medication has extended contact with the skin.
- They are inexpensive and widely accessible.

The disadvantages of hydrocarbon bases:

- If applied for an extended period of time, it may cause the skin to get macerated and then water logged.
- It keeps body heat in, which could result in an uncomfortable warmth.
- Due of their stickiness, they are unpleasant to apply and can contaminate clothing.
- Incorporating water into hydrocarbon bases only in low concentrations (less then 5%) and with careful mixing.

ii. Absorption bases :

Small amounts of water are present in absorption bases. Compared to hydrocarbon bases, they offer considerably less emollient qualities. Absorption bases are similar to hydrocarbon bases in that they are hydrophobic, making them difficult to wash off the skin. These can either be water in oil emulsions that make it possible to incorporate an aqueous phase without phase inversion or cracking, or they can be non-aqueous formulations to which an aqueous phase can be added to create a water in Oil (w/o) emulsion. The essential characteristics of water in oil emulsions and non-emulsified bases that are important for the creation of ointments and pastes.

(a) Non - emulsified bases :

These formulations are water-addable hydrophobic substances. They aid in the skin penetration of drugs that are soluble in oil. After application, a film is created that provides occlusion and hence emollient qualities, however these are less occlusive than hydrocarbon bases. A sterol-based emulsifying agent plus one or more paraffins are frequently used to make non-emulsified bases. Examples of emulsifying agents that are commonly used in absorption bases: lanolin (wool fat) ,hydrous lanolin, lanolin alcohols (wool alcohols) , beeswax (yellow/white).

(b) Water in oil (w/o) emulsions :

It has the ability to absorb more water while still performing in a same manner comparable to that of non-emulsified bases in terms of occlusion, spreading qualities, etc. This type of ointment base frequently contains an excipient that is composed of around 25%–30% water and 70–75% hydrous lanolin. To create a base that can accommodate the later addition of an aqueous phase, it is combined with paraffin and oils. The amount of water in bases made with hydrous lanolin is significant. For reference, Oily Cream BP is a water-in-oil emulsion ointment basis made of wool alcohols (50% w/w) and water (50% w/w).

Advantages of absorption bases:

- They facilitate the skin penetration of oil-soluble medications.
- They are good emollients but less occlusive.
- They spread more readily.
- They work with the majority of medications
- They have decent thermal stability.
- They have a large water or aqueous material absorption capacity.
- The base can be employed either in their emulsified or anhydrous form.

Disadvantages of absorption bases:

- Despite their hydrophilicity, absorption bases are challenging to clean.

iii. Water soluble bases :

To achieve the necessary ointment consistency, water-soluble bases are typically produced using combinations of polyethylene glycol with differing molecular weights (macrogols). Polyethylene glycol (PEG) is a combination of polycondensation products of ethylene oxide and water. It basic formula is :

CH_2 OH (CH_2 OCH), CH_2 OH

An example of a water-soluble base is polyethylene glycol (PEG) ointment National Formulary (NF). One can create a product with an ointment-like consistency by mixing waxy and liquid PEG in the right amounts. The mixture of 65% PEG 300 and 35% PEG 4000 is appropriate for use as an ointment base (Macrogol ointment BPC). Tragacanth, gelatin, sodium alginate, pectin, silica gel, magnesium-aluminum silicate, cellulose derivatives, and bentonite are a few more materials that are utilized as water-soluble bases. Although they swell as water is absorbed, many compounds are actually not water soluble.

Advantages of water soluble bases:

- They can be very quickly removed from the skin and are easily miscible with tissue exudates because they are water soluble.
- They facilitate effective skin absorption.
- They are effective solvents. Several water-soluble dermatological drugs, like salicylic acid, sulfonamides, sulphur etc. are soluble in this base.
- They are not greasy.
- They don't hydrolyze, become rancid, or promote microbial development.
- They work well with a variety of dermatological medications.

Disadvantages of water soluble bases:

- Water absorption is constrained; macrogols dissolve at around 5% water content.
- They are less bland than paraffin because they are hygroscopic.
- Reduction in the antibacterial activity of several substances, such as phenols, hydroxybenzoates, and quaternary compounds.
- Impact of solvent on bakelite and polyethylene containers and closures.

iv. Water-miscible bases :

In contrast to hydrocarbon and absorption bases, water removable bases can include a significant amount of aqueous phase with the help of proper emulsifying agents. These bases' hydrophilic properties make them simple to remove from skin. For tropical applications, these are used to formulate oil-in-water emulsions. Emulsifying ointment, Cetrimide emulsifying ointment, and Cetomacrogol emulsifying ointment are the names given by the British Pharmacopoeia to describe the three types of water-miscible/removable bases. Each of them contains 30% w/w anionic, cationic, or non-ionic emulsifying wax, 50% w/w white soft paraffin, and 20% w/w liquid paraffin.

- Anionic emulsifying wax:

This waxy solid, such as Aqueous Cream BP, which includes 10% w/w anionic emulsifying wax, can be used to create an oil in water emulsion when combined with a paraffin base. 90 g of cetostearyl alcohol, 10 g of sodium lauryl sulphate, and 4 ml of distiled water required to form anionic emulsifying wax.

- Non-ionic emulsifying wax:

This product, also known as Cetomacrogol Emulsifying Wax BP, is made up of 200 g of cetomacrogol 1000 and 800 g of cetostearyl alcohol.

- Cationic emulsifying wax:

Also known as Cetrimide Emulsifying Wax BP. 100 g of cetrimide and 900 g of cetostearyl alcohol make up Cationic Emulsifying Wax BP.

Advantages of water miscible bases:

- They may hold huge amounts of water.
- They don't have occlusivity.
- They are simple to remove from clothing and skin. They can also be easily put to and taken off of hair.
- Less interference with the skin's natural processes.
- They have good aesthetic appeal.

2. **Creams :**

In contrast to translucent ointments, creams have an opaque look and are viscous semisolid emulsion systems. The cream's rheological characteristics and thickness depend on whether it is w/o or o/w. Oil in Water (O/W) creams that have been properly formulated are a sophisticated drug delivery method that are good in appearance and the touch after application. O/W creams are rinsable and non-greasy in nature. They work well topically and are thought to be especially well suited for use on oozing injury.

3. **Pastes :**

Pastes are differ from ointments, that they generally contain a large quantity of finely crushed solids like starch, zinc oxide, calcium carbonate, etc. Due to the presence of these substances they generally get relatively thick and stiff than the ointments but are less greasy than ointments.

Since pastes are stiff they don't melt at ordinary temperature therefore forming and holding a protective coating over the surface to which they're applied. They can be applied to the affected part with the help of a spatula or they may be spread on any of the dressing material and also applied. They aren't removed for quite a long time. The pastes aren't suitable for use to the hair because they're actually tough to remove from there.

4. **Gels (jellies) :**

Gels are semisolid preparations in which a liquid phase is restrained inside a three-dimensional polymeric matrix with a high level of physical or chemical cross-linking (which may contain both natural and synthetic gum). Essentially, gels are hydrated form of insoluble drugs in aqueous colloidal suspensions. Jellies are non-greasy, clear or translucent semisolid gels applied topically on the skin.

Gels are used for drug antiseptic or spermicidal purposes, lubrication. Other uses for gels include serving as carriers for spermicidal chemicals that are administered intra vaginally with diaphragms as an additional method of contraception. It is also used to lubricate surgical hands, catheters, and rectal thermometers. Since jellies contain carbohydrates and lot of water as base thus they have tendency to microbial growth so they must be suitably stored .

For the preparation of jellies there are some generally used gelling agents - tragacanth, starch, sodium alginate, pectin, gelatin, methyl cellulose, carbomer, polyvinyl alcohols, etc.

5. **Plasters :**

Plasters are solid or semi-solid substances applied to the skin for protection, mechanical support or enhance the intimate contact between the drug molecules and the skin. For the preparation of plaster the mass is melted and the drug is added. After that the mixed mass is rolled into sticks and spread upon cloth, paper, linen or plastic. They're cut into different shapes according to the requirements.

The mostly used plasters are back plasters, chest plasters, breast plasters, kidney plasters, and corn plasters. The most commonly used preparation of this type is Self-adhesive plaster (or tape). It doesn't need warming before using it because it sticks to the skin at body temperature.

6. **Poultices :** Poultices seem to be paste-like medications applied externally to relieve inflammation because they effectively hold heat. After heating, the preparation is thickly placed on a dressing and applied to the affected area as hot as the patient can tolerate.

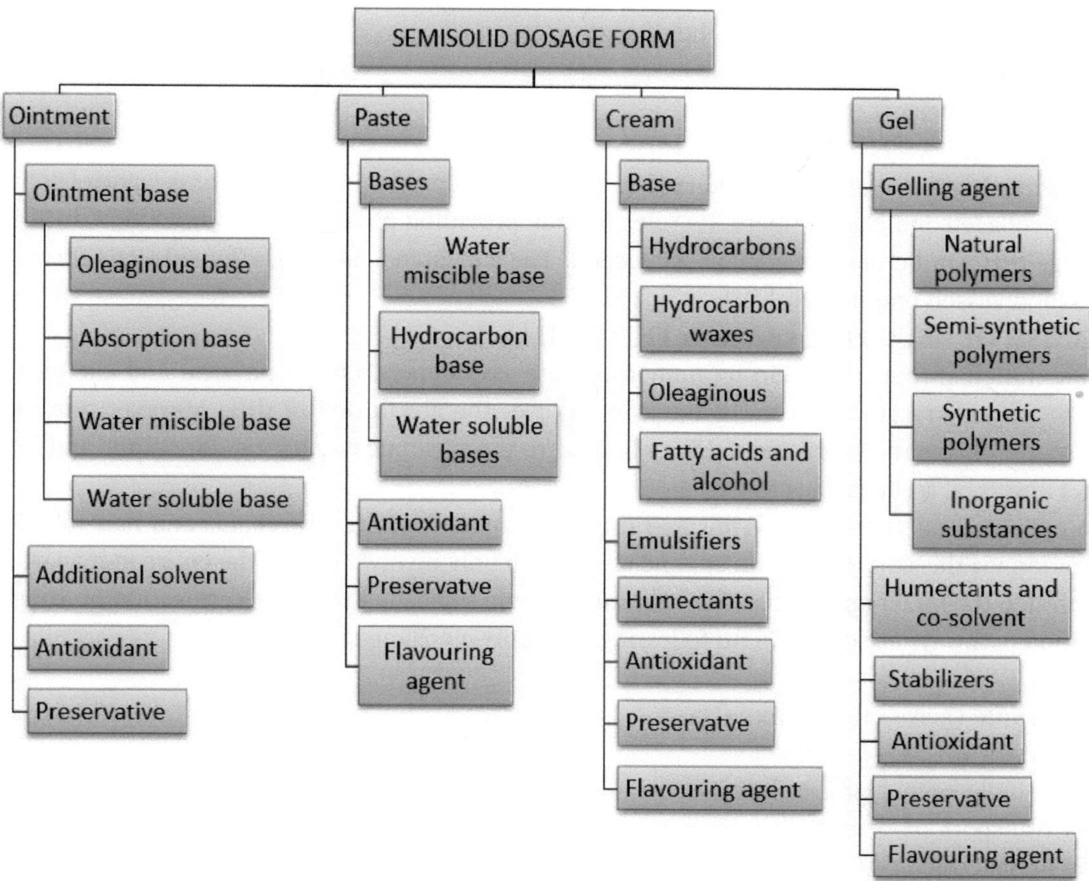

Fig .1.2 Classification of Semisolid Dosage Form

SKIN ANATOMY

In arrangement to understand mechanism or process of dermal penetration of medicines or drugs, one should endure the anatomy of skin. The skin acts as a strong barrier to materials, enabling just a minimal amount of medicine to penetrate it over time. The surface area of human skin is 1.8 to 2.0 m^2, which is largest organ in the body. The skin protect the body from many environmental factors and regulates water and heat loss from body .

Skin has four main layers : stratum corneum, epidermis, dermis, and subcutaneous tissues .

1. **Stratum corneum :**

The stratum corneum, commonly referred to as the "horny layer," is the skin's outermost layer and is roughly 10 mm thick when dry. It has roughly 10–25 rows of - lying dead, keratinized cells, referred as corneocytes. Although flexible, it is largely impermeable. The primary resistance against drug penetration is the stratum corneum.

2. **Epidermis :**

The epidermis layer lies below the stratum corneum and ranges in thickness from 0.06 mm on the eyelids to 0.8 mm on the palms. The stratum lucidum, stratum granulosum, stratum spinosum, and stratum basal are among its layers.

3. **Dermis :**

The dermis is made up of connective tissue mayrix that includes blood vessels, lymph vessels, and nerve tissue. Dermis layer thickness ranges from 3 to 5 mm. The continuous blood flow regulates body temperature and supplies oxygen and nutrients to the skin, among other things.

4. **Subcutaneous tissues :**

The subcutaneous tissue, generally referred to as the hypodermis, is made up of a layer of lobulated fat cells connected by collagen and elastin fibers. Its roles include providing physical shock protection, heat insulation, and energy storage that can be made accessible as needed. The subcutaneous tissues/hypodermis serve to connect the skin to the blood vessels and nerves.

MECHANISM OF DRUG PENETRATION THROUGH SKIN

Drug penetration through the skin by numerous pathways depends upon physical and chemical properties of the drug. The upper stratum corneum of the skin opposes the absorption of drug however presence of different absorption routes enable the entry and delivery of drug to the systemic circulation .Lipophilic and hydrophilic both drugs are get absorbed from various routes.

Diffusion of the drug via the epidermis and the skin's appendages (sweat glands and hair follicles) constitutes drug penetration via the skin. These skin appendages, which only involve 0.1% of the entire human skin, create shunt pathways through the intact epidermis. The stratum corneum typically limits the permeation of drugs through skin. Skin absorption pathways are divided into following transport mechanism :

1. **Epidermal route (across the intact SC) :**

(a) Trans-cellular route (intra-cellular) :

It means transport of drug molecules across epithelial cell membrane. It encompasses the endocytosis and transcytosis of macromolecules, the active transport of ionic and polar components, passive transport of tiny molecules. Because of the extremely poor permeability through corneocytes and the requirement to partition multiple times from the more hydrophilic corneocytes into the lipid Intercellular layers with in the stratum corneum and vice versa, the transcellular route is not often considered as the preferred method of dermal invasion. When a penetration enhancer is used the transcellular pathway can gain significance, for eg. via altering the keratin structure urea increases the permeability of the comeocytes.

(b) Para-cellular route (inter-cellular) :

This pathway involves the movement of molecules inside or outside of cells. The cells include tight junctions or similar situations. The partition coefficient (log k) has a specific role in determining a permeate's primary pathway . Hydrophilic medicines preferentially partition into the intercellular domain names while lipophilic medications permeate (o/w log k>2) the stratum comeum by the intracellular pathway. Due to the high diffusion coefficient of the majority of medications within the lipid bilayer, the intercellular route is taken into account to produce significantly faster absorption..

2. **Trans-follicular/shunt pathway (along the skin appendages) :**

Drug transport through apocrine sweat glands, eccrine sweat glands, and hair follicles with their accompanying sebaceous glands is part of drug penetration through the skin appendageal channel. Shunt pathway is the label given to these routes because they avoid penetration via stratum corneum. Due to the trans-follicular pathway's small area (about 0.1% of the total skin area), it is thought to be of less importance. In contrast, the early stages of a skin absorption process and the invasion of large hydrophilic substances and ions through the appendages may both have a significant effect.

Skin absorption pathways :

Penetration of drug through skin involve some following steps :

1. Penetration : The entery of drug into a specific skin layer .
2. Partitioning : From outermost layer of the skin - stratum corneum into the aqueous viable epidermis.
3. Diffusion : Diffusion into the upper dermis from the viable epidermis.
4. Permeation : Drug molecule permeat from one layer into another.
5. Absorption : Uptake of drug into the local capillary network and then into the systemic circulation.

Generally, diffusion of compounds across the stratum corneum is described by Fick's first law (Fick's Law of Diffusion). Law states that the " Flux (rate of transfer per unit area) of a compound (J, mass/cm^2 per second) at a given time and position is proportional to the differential concentration change dC over a differential distance dx (i.e. the concentration gradient dC/dx) ".

$$J = -D\frac{dC}{d}$$

The negative (-) sign in the equation shows that net flux is moving in the direction of decreasing the activity of thermodynamic and that also can represent by concentration. By combining a differential mass balance in a membrane with Fick's first law, Fick's second law (describing concentration within a membrane) is derived. While considering the skin, assume that the drug is not metabolized, the drug doesn't bind, and its diffusion coefficient doesn't differ with position or composition.

$$\frac{dC}{dt} = \frac{Dd^2C}{dx^2}$$

Fick's first law, which treats the different layers of the skin as pseudo-homogeneous membranes, can be used to characterize the diffusion processes in these layers. The flux at steady state (Jss) ,for a membrane of thickness h is given by :

$$Jss = \frac{D(C_1 - C_2)}{h}$$

where,

C_1 and C_2 - concentrations of the chemical in the membrane at the two faces (ie. at x = 0 and x = h)

D - effective diffusion coefficient

h – thickness of membrane

FACTORS INFLUENCING DERMAL PENETRATION OF DRUGS :

Biological factors :

1. **Skin condition :**

Drugs penetration through helthy skin is difficult, while acids and alkalis damage barrier cells, which makes penetration easier. Molecules flow more easily when mixtures of polar and non-polar solvents (such chloroform and methanol) are used to dissolve the lipid portion. With loss of stratum corneum , disease alters skin condition, or skin inflamed therefore increases the permeability.

2. **Skin age :**

The skin of children and elderly once is more permeable than adult tissue. Children's larger surface area per unit body weight makes them more susceptible to the effects of hazardous medications and chemicals; as a result, powerful topical steroids can have fatal side effects.

3. **Blood flow :**

An increase in blood flow increases the concentration gradient across the skin and shortens the time a penetrant stays in the dermis.

4. **Regional skin site :**

Variations in permeability depend on the the density of skin appendages and on the consistency and nature of stratum corneum. Absorption changes with volunteer, site and substance. Permeabilities depend on thickness of the tissue and stratum corneum.

Because of the thin layers of stratum corneum, the postauricular skin (i.e., the skin behind the ear) uses the hyoscine Transderm system.Compared to other body regions, the skin on the face is more porous.

5. **Skin metabolism :**

Skin can only metabolize upto 5% of toplical drugs. It has advantage to prodrugs. The skin metabolizes chemical carcinogens, steroid hormones, and some drugs.

6. Species difference :

To assess percutaneous absorption animals such as mice, rats and rabbits are used, but as compare to human skin, their skins have more hair follicles and they lack sweat glands. However, using human skin is the best way to get better skin penetration statistics.

7. **Stratum corneum layer :**

Penetration of drug increases with increased thinness of stratum corneum layer. On face the stratum corneum layer is thinnest and thickest on soles and palms .

8. **Skin hydration :**

When skin get saturated due to water, the tissue swells, softens and wrinkles, and the hydration of the stratum corneum makes it more permeable. Lotions or dusting powder increases the surface area for evaporation and dries the skin . Drug penetration increases by hydration .

Physicochemical factors :

1. **Solubility :**

Moderately lipid soluble molecules penetrates directly across the stratum corneum and highly lipid soluble molecules penetrates through hair follicles .

2. **Temperature and pH :**

For significant temperature fluctuations, the rate of substance penetration into human skin can vary by a factor of 10. The temperature and permeability of the skin are increased by occlusive vehicles.

Only unionized molecules, according to the pH-partition theory, can easily traverse lipid membranes. Depending on the pH and the pKa or pKb values, weak acids and bases dissociate to variable degrees. The pH range of 3-9, is not harmful to the stratum corneum.

3. **Diffusion coefficient :**

The state of the matter in the medium affects a molecule's rate of diffusion. The diffusion coefficient is higher in gases than it is in liquids. In compacted to matrix of the stratum corneum in the skin, the diffusion coefficient reaches its lowest value. The nature of the drug, the diffusion medium, and their interactions all affect a drug's diffusion coefficient in a topical vehicle.

4. **Drug concentration :**

The concentration gradient that passes across the barrier directly affects drug permeability and solute flux. The maximum flux is produced by saturated donor solution and Fick's law for drug penetration. The effective partition coefficient is affected by pH changes, complex formation, the presence of surfactants, micelles, or cosolvents, among other factors.

5. **Partition coefficient :**

The flow of medication through the stratum corneum is determined in part by the partition coefficient. Drugs that are ($K>1$) oil soluble and ($K<1$) water soluble. Saturated medication solutions are created by mixing polar solvents, including water and propylene glycol, and this increases the gradient of concentration across the stratum corneum. Surfactants disrupt the stratum corneum's intercellular lipid packing and increase penetration. Drug absorption may be aided by the development of a drug compound that raises the partition coefficient.

6. **Molecular weight, size and shape :**

The relationship between absorption and molecular weight is inverse. The skin's surface can be easily penetrated by molecules up to 400 daltons in weight. Smaller molecules can enter the body more quickly than larger ones. Because molecular form is correlated with the partition coefficient, it is challenging to ascertain its impact.

Vehicles :

Vehicles increases the penetration of drug by penetrating the epidermis layer, by the increase in degree of the stratum corneum, by altering the permeability of the skin, or by good contact with the skin .

Additives :

Surfactants e.g., quaternary ammonium compounds, alkali soaps etc are used to enhances the penetration because they are surface active agents which reduces the surface tension. Humectants e.g. glycerine, polyethylene glycol etc. are used to increase the solubility of active ingredients. Penetration enhancers like ethanol, oleic acid etc. are used to improve penetration.

PREPARATION OF OINTMENTS, PASTES, CREAMSAND GEL

1. **OINTMENTS:**

Ointments are uniform, semi-solid substances that are applied externally to the skin or mucous membranes. When some degree of occlusion is desired, they are used as emollients or for the application of active ingredients to the skin for protective, therapeutic, or preventive purposes. To create preparations that are immiscible, miscible, or emulsifiable with skin secretions, ointments are made with hydrophilic, hydrophobic, or water-emulsifying bases. They can also be made from hydrocarbons (Tatty), water-miscible, water-soluble bases or water miscible , absorption.

Ointments' ideal features are:

- It should be grittiness-free and smooth.
- Physically and chemically stable is required.
- At body temperature, it should melt or become soft and be simple to apply.
- The basis must not be therapeutic and must not be imitation.
- The medication needs to be evenly distributed throughout the base after being finely split.

The different types of ointments:

Following are the categories of ointments according to their therapeutic applications and their penetration:

According to therapeutic application :

- Antibacterial ointments:

Used to eliminate bacteria. Examples include neomycin, bacitracin, and chlortetracycline.

- Anti-fungal creams:

It is used to eliminate fungi. Examples include benzoic acid, salicylic acid, nystatin, etc.

- Anti-inflammatory ointments:

Used to treat allergic, inflammatory, and urticaria disorders. Examples include fluocinolone acetonid, betamethasone valerate, triamcinolone acetonide, hydrocortisone and its acetate etc.

- Antipruritic ointments:

Used to soothe itchiness. Examples include coal tar and benzocaine.

- Astringent ointments:

Utilized to shrink or constrict skin cells or mucous membranes by precipitating proteins from their surface. When used topically, they dry harden, and the skin is protected. They are used to treat minor wounds, allergies, dermatitis, stretch marks, bug bites, and other skin irritations. They also lessen bleeding from minor abrasions. Examples: zinc oxide, calamine, tannic acid, acetic acid etc.

- Antiecrematous ointments:

Intended to stop coding and excretion from the skin's vesicles. Hydrocortisone, ichthamol, salicylic acid, coal tar, sulphur, etc. are a few examples.

- Kertolytic ointments:

Used to soften the horny layer or stratum corneum of skin. Some examples are sulphur, salicylic acid, and resorcinol.

- Counter-irritant ointments:

Applied topically to the skin, which lessens or relieves a distinct irritation or intense pain. Examples include oleoresin, methyl salicyla lodine, and capsicum.

- Antidandruff ointments:

Used as a dandruff remedy. Examples include cetimida and salicylic acid.

- Ointment for psoriasis treatment:

Used as psoriasis treatment. Examples include salicylic acid, diathranol b, corticosteroids, and coal tar.

- Parasiticide ointments:

Used to eliminate or prevent live infestations, such as lice and scabies. Examples include sulphur, hexachloride, and benzyl benzoate.

- Ointments for protection:

Used to shield skin from elements like moisture, air, sunlight. Example include zinc oxide, calamine, titanium dioxide etc.

According to penetration :

- Epidermic Ointments:

These creams are made with the intention to give or produce local effect and action on the skin's surface. They serve as parasiticides, antiseptics, and protective agents.

- Endodermic Ointments:

These ointments are made to allow the skin-penetrating medications to be released. They serve as emollients, stimulants, and local irritants and are only partially absorbed.

- Diadermic Ointments:

These ointments are designed to release medications that penetrate the skin and have an impact throughout the body.

Advantages of Ointments :

- They prevent the drug's first pass metabolism.
- They offer methods for applying medication site-specifically to the injured section, preventing unwanted exposure to the medication outside of its intended use and preventing side effects.

- They work well as dose forms for medications with a bitter taste.
- Convenient for oral administration specially for unconscious patients.
- In comparison to liquid dose forms, they are easier to handle and more chemically stable.

Disadvantages of Ointments :

- These greasy semisolid formulations leave stains and are less used cosmetically.
- Application with a fingertip has the potential to contaminate the product or may cause irritate the skin.
- Ointments are heavier to handle than solid dose forms.
- Although semisolids offer greater dose flexibility, dose accuracy is based on the quantity to be applied being applied uniformly.
- Less stable in terms of physico-chemistry than solid dose forms

Ointment preparation techniques :

The active ingredients are either mixed with the desired basis to create ointments, or the base and active ingredient are melted together.

1. **Fusion method:**

It is necessary to melt the solid elements that make up an ointment base, such as white beeswax, cetyl alcohol, stearyl alcohol, stearic acid, hard paraffin, etc. There are two ways to melt things:

a. Method-I:

The components are melted in decreasing order of their melting points, starting with the component having the higher m.p., then moving on to the component with the next melting point, and so on. When the materials are melted, the medication is gently poured into the mixture and properly mixed until a homogeneous result. This will prevent low melting point materials from overheating.

b. Method-II:

All of the parts are separated up and then melted together. Because the materials with lower melting points act as solvents on the other ingredients, the maximum temperature reached is lower than as compare with Method-1, and the process took less time.

Precautions:

- By grinding waxy ingredients (such as beeswax, wool alcohols, hard-paraffin, higher fatty alcohols, and emulsifying waxes), stirring while melting, and dropping the dish as far into the water bath as possible so that the most surface area is heated, the melting time can be decreased.
- Some materials, such as wool fats and wool alcohols, oxidise to produce a discoloured surface that needs to be cleaned prior to use.
- The ingredients should be mixed once they have melted until the ointment has cooled, being careful not to produce localised cooling, for eg by using a cold spatula or stirrer. putting the dish on a cold surface (such a plastic bench top) or moving the ointment to a cold container before it has had time to set completely.
- After the ointment has started to thicken, vigorous stirring promotes excessive aeration and should be avoided.
- Many ingredients in ointment bases pick up dirt during storage since they are oily, which can be visible after melting. This is taken out of the melt by passing it through muslin that is held by a warm strainer, allowing it to settle, and then decanting the supernatant. The clarified liquid is collected in a second hot basin in both cases.

- If the product becomes granular after cooling because components with high melting points have separated, it should be re-melted with the least amount of heat, then mixed and cooled again.

Method:

Cetostearyl alcohol with hard paraffin on a water bath. Until all the materials are melted, wool fat and white soft paraffin are combined and blended. If necessary, it can be decanted or filtered, mixed until cold, and then stored in an appropriate container.

Uses:

Simple ointment made with white soft paraffin should be used as a base for white ointments, and if it is made with yellow soft paraffin, it should be used as a base for coloured ointments, unless otherwise indicated. Wool fat has an emollient effect. It is not easily absorbed on its own, but when combined with sufficient vegetable oil or soft paraffin, it creates a cream that penetrates the skin and aids in the absorption of therapeutically active ingredients. As a stiffening agent, hard paraffin is used. The emollient qualities of ointments are enhanced by cetostearyl alcohol.

Medicated ointment by fusion method:

Fine powdered particles that are fully or partially soluble should be added to the molten base at a very low temperature and stirred until the mixture cools. Just as the base is thickening, at about 40°C, liquids like methyl salicylate and coal tar solutions, as well as semi-solids like ichthamol, should be added. It is easier to add a solid ingredient in solution when it is soluble in a liquid ingredient, such as menthol in methyl salicylate. When the base begins to thicken, the insoluble solids (calamine, starch, and zinc oxide) should be added in small amounts while stirring through a 180 um screen. It is important to avoid sedimentation. A less amount of the product's liquid paraffin or fixed oil can be used to loosen the powder before adding it to the base to create a smoother final result.

Example: Salicylic Ointment BP : Salicylic acid 2% w/w and Wool alcohol ointment q.s.

Wool Alcohol Ointment : Wool alcohols 60g, Hard paraffin 240g, White soft paraffin 100 g, Liquid paraffin 600g

Method:

Salicylic acid is added to the molten base while the wool alcohol ointment BP, the preparation's base, is continuously stirred until it cools. White soft paraffin, which is colourless, is utilised in this procedure to make wool alcohol ointment.

Use : For the treatment of psoriasis and hyperkeratotic diseases

2. <u>Trituration technique :</u>

This technique can be used with a base or a less amount of liquid. Solids are sieved (# 250, 180, #125) after being finely crushed. A small amount of the base is used to triturate the powder after it has been placed on an ointment slab (Levigation). For this, a steel spatula with a long, broad blade is utilised. Additional amounts of the base are added and triturated with this until the medication is combined with the base. Ingredients in liquid form are added last. Before adding additional in the same manner, a small amount of liquid is put into a depression in the ointment to prevent loss due to splashing. Splashing is easier to regulate in a mortar than it is on an ointment slab.

Method:

Benzoic acid and salicylic acid are sieved via No. 180 sieves. On the ointment slab, they are combined with a little amount of base, levitated until smooth, and then gently diluted.

Use : For the treatment of skin fungus infections

Marketed products:

500 g of Whitfield ointment, a compound benzoic acid ointment, is available from Bell's Healthcare. Fungalin (Chemist Laboratories Ltd.), Sibex (Elixir Pharmaceuticals Ltd.), Benzalic (Central Pharmaceuticals Ltd.), and G-Benzosal (Gonoshasthaya) .

Example: Salicylic Acid Sulphur Ointment BPC

Salicylic acid BP 30 g, Precipitated sulphur BP 30 g, Oily cream BP 940g.

Method: Trituration method

Use: To treat acne and dandruff

3. <u>Chemical Reaction :</u>

Many ointments exhibit chemical reactions while being made.

a. **Free iodine-containing ointment :**

Due to the production of molecular complexes like KI, I_2, $Kl.2I_2$, $KI.3I_2$, etc., iodine is only minimally soluble in most fats and oils but very readily soluble in concentrated aqueous potassium iodide solution. These solutions may be included in bases for ointments that absorb moisture. Cattle with ringworm are treated with strong lodine ointment from the British Veterinary Pharmacopoeia (B.Vet.C). It has iodine that is free. When treating human rheumatic disorders, these ointments were once recommended as counter irritants, but they were unpopular since they stain the skin a dark red shade and because of improper storage, the water evaporates and the iodine crystals hurt the skin, consequently, glycerol was occasionally utilized in place of water to dissolve the iodine-potassium iodide combination.

Example: Strong lodine Ointment B.Vet.C.

Method:

Mix KI with water. Iodine should be mixed in. Melt yellow soft paraffin separately in a water bath. A 40°C cooling occurs on the melted substance. Once the mixture has melted, gradually add the iodine solution while constantly stirring it until you have an uniform mass. Bring to room temperature before packing.

Use: Cattle ringworm.

b. Combination iodine-containing ointment :

Iodine is absorbed by fixed oils and many vegetable and animal fats, where it binds with the double bonds of the ingredients that are unsaturated.

$CH_3 (CH_2)_7 CH = CH(CH_2)_7.COOH + I_2 = CH_3(CH_2)_7.CHI.CHI.(CH_2)_7COOH$

Oleic acid di-iodo stearic acid

Example: Non-staining lodine Ointment BPC 1968

Methods :

- Iodine should be mixed thoroughly in a glass mortar before being mixed with oil in a conical flask with a glass cap.
- In a water bath, heat the oil to 50°C while stirring constantly. Heating should continue until the brown tone turns greenish-black, which could take many hours.
- 40°C soft paraffin warming. Mix thoroughly before adding iodized oil. Continued heating should be avoided to prevent the deposition of a resinous material.
- Put the preparation in a heated, wide-mouthed glass bottle that is amber in colour. Without more stirring, let it cool.

Uses : Antiseptic and irritant-blocking.

2. PASTES :

Pastes are uniform, semi-solid preparations that are distributed in a suitable base and have high concentrations of insoluble powdered materials (often not less than 20%). Ointments with a significant proportion of powder dispersed in a fatty base are short paste. Because there are so many powdered constituents in pastes, they are typically less greasy, more absorbent, and stiffer in texture than ointments. Some pastes, like hydrated pectin, are made of a single phase, whilst other pastes are made of a thick, hard substance that does not flow at body temperature. The pastes ought to stick to the skin well. They frequently provide a shielding layer that regulates water evaporation.

Characteristics of paste over ointments:

- In general, pastes contain 50% or more of finely powdered particles. Therefore, they are frequently stiffer than ointments.

- Pastes are porous because they include powder, allowing sweat to escape. Pastes with a hydrocarbon base are less macerating than ointments with a comparable base because the powder absorbs exudates.
- Pastes stick effectively to the skin when applied, providing a thick coating that soothes, protects, and treats raw, irritated surfaces. This coating also lessens the damage caused by scratching in itching disorders like persistent eczema. Pastes are relatively simple to contain to the sick areas, while ointments, which are often less viscous, have a tendency to transfer to the healthy skin, which might cause hypersensitive reactions if the preparations contain a potent medication like diathranol.
- Though less oily than ointments, pastes lack aesthetic appeal because their effectiveness depends on maintaining a thick surface layer.
- Because they are difficult to remove from the hair, the majority of the pastes are ineffective for treating scalp disorders.

Paste preparation :

Hydrocarbon base, water miscible base, and water soluble base are bases that are used to prepare pastes similarly to ointment base. Other additives are identical to ointments. Pastes can also be made through the fusion and trituration processes. When the base is solid or semisolid in composition, the fusion process is used. When the base is liquid or semisolid, the trituration method is used.

i. **Pastes prepared by fusion method :**

Method I :

Wax for emulsification is 70 °C melted on a petri dish. Coal tar should be added in weighed amounts to melted wax. Melt the yellow soft paraffin separately. With constant stirring, add half of the melted yellow soft paraffin to the coal tar and wax mixture above. Once homogenous, add the remaining portion of melted yellow soft paraffin. Allow to cool to 30°C, then add the starch and zinc oxide (which had previously been put through sieve number 180) while stirring continuously. Stir until the mixture becomes cool.

Method-II:

Mix thoroughly and stir until just setting after melting emulsifying wax and yellow soft paraffin together. Coal tar is added after mixing zinc oxide powder with the melted wax in the previous step on a warm ointment slab using levigation. The chance of overheating is eliminated by this technique.

Examples of fusion method is Zinc and Coal tar Paste (White's Tar Paste)

Use: It is used to treatment of psoriasis and eczema.

ii. **Pastes prepared by fusion and trituration method :**

Method:

Starch and zinc oxide are crushed through sieve 180. Melt white soft paraffin on a water bath separately. Add the necessary amount of powder to a heated mortar and well blend in some melted white soft paraffin. As the mixture cools, gently add the remaining base.

Use: For the treatment of skin issues like psoriasis and eczema. Sun protection is possible.

Example is Compound Zinc Paste BP.

3. CREAMES :

Creams are opaque emulsion systems that are homogeneous, semi-solid formulations. Whether an emulsion is water-in-oil (w/o) or oil-in-water (o/w), as well as on the type of solids in the internal phase, determines the consistency and rheological characteristics. In cases where an occlusive effect is not required, creams are applied to the skin or specific mucous membranes for preventive, therapeutic, or protective purposes. The most popular use of the word "cream" is to refer to smooth, aesthetically pleasing dishes.

Preparation of creams :

Wax and other oils are used as the oil phase and water as the aqueous phase since creams are emulsions with fatty bases. When making cream, different emulsifiers are added to create emulsions, or soap is created when fatty acids and alkalis react, acting as an emulsifying agent.

1. Preparation of oil phase:

Ingredients in the form of flakes or powder are scattered in mineral oil or silicone oil after being dry mixed in advance. Some ingredients might need to be heated in order to melt.

2. Hydration of aqueous phase ingredients:

In a different vessel, emulsifiers, thickeners, and stabilisers are diluted with water. Heating can be necessary to hasten hydration.

3. Forming the emulsion:

To create the emulsion, the two phases are vigorously agitated while being mixed at the same temperature.

4. Distribution of the active component:

In order to enhance production and product effectiveness, the active ingredient, which frequently makes up a small fraction of the formulation, must be properly disseminated. In order for the internal phase to solidify, o/w creams are often prepared at a high temperature and then cooled to room temperature. A w/o cream's semi-solid consistency can be attributed to the nature of the exterior phase.

a. **Oily creams (w/o) :**

These creams are hydrophobic, typically anhydrous, and barely absorb water. They contain emulsifying agents (like monoglycerides, sorbitan esters, and wool fat). The term "oily cream" also applies to hydrous ointment. Although it isn't an active component but, this acts as a moisturiser by coating the skin's surface in oil to stop water from evaporating. It is an extremely oily moisturiser. Water and wool alcohol ointment are combined or mixed with phenoxyethanol as an antibacterial preservative.

Example: Hydrous ointment BP or Oily cream .

Use: For all cases of extremely dry skin, including eczema and dermatitis.

b. Aqueous creams (o/w) :

These hydrophilic creams have water-miscible bases in them. Additionally they contain o/w emulsifying agents such as sodium or triethanolamine soaps, sulfated fatty alcohols, and polysorbates, if necessary with w/o emulsifying agents. These creams are miscible with skin secretions.

Example: Aqueous, cetrimide, and cetomacrogol creams.

Use: Emollients are used to treat the symptoms of dry skin disorders.

c. Cosmetic creams :

These creams, which come in w/o and o/w varieties, are utilised as cosmetic preparations.

Examples include all-purpose, baby, barrier, bleaching, cleansing, cold, hair, hand, and disappearing creams.

Use: Foundation cream to hold face powder and moisturiser.

d. Medicated creams :

To carry medications, either w/o or o/w kind of cream is used as the base in this type of cream.

Example:

Psoriasis, eczema, and rashes caused by poison oak or poison ivy are all treated with hydrocortisone cream. Creams containing antibiotics are used to treat mild infections and abrasions. creams with antifungal properties used for ringworm, candida intertrigo, or diaper rash. Baby diaper rash and sunburn are both treated with zinc oxide cream.

Use : antifungal lotion

4. GELS :

Gels are typically homogenous, transparent, semi-solid preparations that contain a liquid phase inside of a three-dimensional polymeric matrix with appropriate gelling agents creating physical or occasionally chemical cross-links to the liquid phase. Simply put, gels are semisolid compositions that have liquid dissolved into large or small organic or inorganic molecules.

Due to their ease of manufacture and suitability for drug administration via the epidermal, oral, buccal, ocular, nasal, otic, and vaginal routes, gels are appealing delivery systems. Additionally, they allow for close contact between the medicine and the location of action or absorption.Due to the development of polymer science, gel-based systems are being developed and tested that react to particular biological or environmental cues such pH, temperature, ionic strength, enzymes, antigens, light, magnetic field, ultrasound, and electric current .

Classification of Gels :

1. Hydrophilic gels:

In order to fix the liquid vehicle as the exterior phase, hydrophilic gels‘ interior phase is constructed of a polymer that forms a cogent three-dimensional net-like structure. The solvent molecules are intermolecularly bound to a polymeric net, reducing their mobility and creating a structured system with higher viscosity. Liquid paraffin with polyethylene or fatty oils gelled with colloidal silica, aluminium, or zinc soaps are the typical ingredients in hydrophobic gel (oleogel) bases.

2. Hydrophilic gels:

Water, glycerol, or propylene glycol are typically the raw materials for hydrophilic gel (hydrogel) bases. These liquids are then gelled with appropriate substances such tragacanth, starch, cellulose derivatives, carboxyvinyl polymers, and magnesium aluminum silicates.

3. Non-Aqueous gels:

Propylene glycol dicaprylate/dicaprate was successfully used to create a nonaqueous gel out of ethyl cellulose. The novel nonaqueous gel displayed rheological profiles corresponding to a physically cross-linked three-dimensional gel network and had appropriate mechanical properties for application as a delivery system for topical medications.

4. Organogels:

Numerous organic solvents, including hexadecane, isopropyl myristate, and a variety of vegetable oils, as well as the hydrophobic nonionic surfactant sorbitan monostearate are present. When an organogelator is dissolved or dispersed in a hot solvent, an organic solution or dispersion is created, which, when cooled, settles to the gel state.

5. Amphiphilic gels:

By combining the liquid phase, such as liquid sorbitan esters or polysorbate, with the solid gelator, such as sorbitan monostearate or sorbitan monopalmitate, and heating the mixture to 60 °C to form an isotropic clear sol phase, it is possible to create amphiphilic gels. The clear isotropic sol phase can then be cooled to room temperature to create an opaque semisolid. The majority of the amphiphilic gel microstructures were made up of groups of tubules of gelator molecules that had gathered after the sol phase had cooled, creating a 3D network throughout the continuous phase. The gels proved to be thermoreversible. With increasing gelator content, the temperature and viscosity of the gelation rose, indicating a more solid gel network. The gels significantly weakened at temperatures close to the skin's surface temperature, enabling topical administration.

6. Thermosensitive sol-gel reversible hydrogels:

They are polymeric solutions that, when exposed to environmental factors like temperature and pH, transition reversibly from sol to gel, forming in-situ hydrogels.

7. Hydrogels:

Hydrogels are gel structures in which an insoluble polymer immobilizes water. Water and a polymeric material that is hydrophilic but not water soluble make up hydrogels. The dry polymer swells and absorbs liquid when it is exposed to water. Either chemical reactions or physical pressures are used to crosslink the polymer strands.

Formulation of gels

Compared to ointments and creams, gels are comparatively simpler to make. Gelling agents, buffers, preservatives, antioxidants, flavoring/sweetening agents, colors, and vehicles are the main ingredients of pharmaceutical gels.

1. Vehicle

The typical solvent or vehicle used in the manufacturing of pharmaceutical gels is purified water. To improve the solubility of the therapeutic agent in the dosage form or (in the case of ethanol) to improve drug penetration across the skin, co-solvents may be employed, such as alcohol, propylene glycol, glycerol, and polyethylene glycol (often polyethylene glycol 400). Pharmaceutical gels may be created utilizing polyhydroxy solvents, such as propylene glycol, glycerol, or polyethylene glycol 400, and polyacidic polymers, such as poly(2-ethylhexylacrylamide), if the medication has poor chemical stability and/or is poorly soluble in water or water-based media.

2. Gel-forming polymers:

A compound made up of repeating units is known as a polymer. The structural network required for the creation of gels is provided by polymers. The following categories apply to bases or polymers that create gels:

i. Natural polymers:

Natural polymers are those that can be produced by living organisms and are present in nature, such as proteins like collagen and gelatine and polysaccharides like agar, tragacanth, pectin, and gum.

ii. Semi synthetic polymers:

These polymers, such as cellulose derivatives like carboxymethyl cellulose, methylcellulose, hydroxypropyl cellulose, and hydroxyethyl cellulose, are primarily generated from natural polymers through chemical modification.

iii. Synthetic polymers:

Synthetic polymers are defined as those created in laboratories.T hese are also known as man-made polymers.For eg. Carbopol 934, Poloxamer, Polyacrylamide and Carbopol 940.

iv. Inorganic substances: Bentonite and Aluminium hydroxide
v. Surfactants: Sebrotearyle alcohol and Brij-96.
vi. Buffers:

Aqueous and hydro-alcoholic based gels may contain buffers (for example, phosphate, citrate) to adjust the pH of the formulation, just as other semisolid formulations.

4. Preservatives :

Preservatives must be added to pharmaceutical gels, and in general, the selection of preservatives is similar to that for ointments and pastes. Certain preservatives, such as parabens and phenolics, should be used with caution since they interact with the hydrophilic polymers used to make gels and lower the concentration of free (antimicrobially active) preservative in the formulation. The original concentration of these preservatives should be increased as a result to make up for this.

5. Antioxidants:

To boost the chemical stability of therapeutic agents that are susceptible to oxidative degradation, antioxidants may be added to the formulation, much like in other semisolid formulations. The type of vehicle needed for making the pharmaceutical gel will determine which antioxidants are used. As a result, water-soluble antioxidants, such as sodium metabisulphite and sodium formaldehyde sulphoxylate, are frequently used, since they are mostly aqueous in nature.

6. Sweetening/flavoring substances:

Only pharmaceutical gels intended for administration into the oral cavity, such as those used to treat infection, inflammation, or ulceration, contain flavoring and sweetening ingredients. The type and concentration of sweetener/flavoring agents chosen to effectively conceal the taste of the drug ingredient depends on the necessary taste as well as the type and concentration.

7. Coloring agents:

FD&C certified colours is used in pharmaceutical gels, as per requirements .

Preparation of gels:

- Fusion technique:

This technique uses a variety of waxy compounds as a gellant in non-polar fluids. Drug is incorporated after waxy materials have melted through fusion and have been slowly mixed into an uniform gel.

- Cold technique :

A mixing container is filled with water that has been cooled to 4–10°C. The gelling ingredient is steadily added while being stirred into the solution. The temperature is kept below 10 °C. The drug is then gradually added in solution form while being gently mixed. When the liquid is immediately moved to a container and warmed to room temperature, it turns into a clear gel.

- Dispersion technique :

Water is mixed with the gelling agent while being stirred at 1200 rpm for 30 minutes. In a non-aqueous solvent with a preservative, the drug is dissolved. The above gel is then gradually added with constant stirring of this solution.

Some principles during gel formation :

1. Flocculation:

Here, gelation is created by adding just the right amount of salt to cause age state precipitation, but not enough to cause full precipitation. In order to prevent localized high precipitant concentrations, rapid mixing is required. For instance, polystyrene in benzene solutions can gel when quickly mixed with the appropriate concentrations of a non-solvent, such as petroleum ether. Salts cause coagulation and gelation when added to hydrophobic solutions, respectively. The behavior of the gels produced by flocculation is thixotropic. Hydrophilic colloids like gelatin, proteins, and acacia are only impacted by high electrolyte concentrations; when the effect is to salt out, the colloidal, gelation doesn't take place.

2. Chemical reaction:

According to this theory, gel is created by the chemical reaction between the solute and solvent. For instance, aluminum hydroxide gel can be created by the reaction of an aluminum salt with sodium carbonate in water, which results in a higher concentration of reactants and the formation of a gel structure. There are a few other instances where the polymeric chain is cross-linked chemically, including PVA, cyanoacrylates with Glycidol ether (Glycidol), toluene diisocyanates (TDI), and methane diphenyl isocyanine (MDI).

3. Thermal variations :

Gelatin is produced when lipophilic colloids (solvated polymers) are heated. In comparison to cold water, several hydrogen formers are more soluble in heat. Gelatin, agar sodium oleate, guar gum, and derivatives of cellulose, are examples of substances that gel as the temperature drops because they have a lower degree of hydration. Some substances, such as cellulose ether, on the other hand, have their water solubility due to hydrogen bonding with the water. These solutions' lower solubility and disrupted hydrogen bonds will result in gelation as the temperature is raised.

Storage and Packing :

The container and closure system, or the packaging material, should be compatible with the formulation's ingredients. The amount of unidentified degradable chemicals may grow due to leaching from the container and closure system. Large-mouth ointment jars, metal or plastic collapsible tubes, tight containers, or other well-closed containers are used to package semisolid preparations. Semisolid preparations need to be kept both in a cool environment to prevent product separation in heat and in tightly closed containers to prevent contamination. Some materials require unique storage conditions, such as protection from light, avoidance of extreme heat, avoidance of direct sunshine, avoidance of bright fluorescent lighting, avoidance of refrigeration, and avoidance of protracted exposure to temperatures above 30°C. Light-sensitive preparations are stored in containers that are opaque or light-resistant when necessary. Various pharmacopoeia specify that the labeling for some ointments and creams must also state the type of base used in addition to the standard labeling requirements for medicinal items (for example, water soluble or water insoluble). For external use only, all topical semisolid dosage forms must bear the supplemental label.

Ideally, well-closed containers should be used to store topical semi-solid dose forms. When maintained at the temperature specified on the label, which should typically not exceed 25°C, the preparation should preserve its medicinal integrity throughout its shelf life. Specific storage guidelines or restrictions are noted in each monograph.

EXCIPIENTS USED IN SEMISOLIDS DOSAGE FORMS

For the preparation of semisolids following excipientsare required : API, Bases, Antioxidants, Penetration enhancer, Emulsifier, Humectants, Buffers, Preservative, Organoleptic agents, Gelling agent, Fragrances.

1. **API :**

Active Pharmaceutical Ingredient (API) are the active ingredient in a drug that produce the required therapeutic effects to the body to cure disease. For example, paracetamol (API) in crocin, it give relief from body ache and fever .

2. **BASES :**

Base is one of the most important component used in formulation of semisolid dosage form. Ointment bases don't simply act as the carriers of the remedies, but they also control the extent of absorption of remedies incorporated in them.

Ideal base characteristics are:

They must be :

- Non-irritating, non-sensitizing, and inert
- Compatible with the pH of skin.
- Decent solvent.
- Excellent emulsifier.
- Non-greasy, easily removed, and emollient.
- At the site of application, the medication releases easily.
- Pharmaceutically sophisticated and stable.

3. **ANTIOXIDANTS :**

Oxygen is a highly reactive atom, that become part of potentially damaging molecules generally called "free radicals." Free radicals are capable of attacking the healthy cells of the body, causing them to lose their structure and function. To counter this an antioxidants are added.

Examples of antioxidants are :

Lipophilic antioxidants : Butylated hydroxyanisole (BHA), butylated hydroxytoluene (BHT), propyl gallate.

Hydrophilic antioxidants : Sodium metabisulphite and sodium sulphite .

4. **PENETRATION ENHANCERS :**

For deep penetration of drug molecules skin can act as a barrier. With the help of penetration enhancers, penetration of the drug through the skin is improved and made easier. Some ideal properties of penetration enhancers are:

- It should be non-toxic.
- It should have rapid onset action for drug used.
- It should be non-irritating and non-allergenic.
- It should have suitable duration of action.

- It should be compatible, physically and chemically with other ingredients.
- It should be less costly and cosmetically acceptable.

eg. Urea, Oleic Acid , Limonene , Geraniol , triethanolamine and etc .

5. **EMULSIFIER :**

An emulsifier (emulgent) is a substance that stabilises an emulsion by increasing its kinetic stability. It must reduce surface tension for proper emulsification. It prevents coalescence. It has the ability to increase the viscosity at a low concentration and it should be effective at low concentration. It is generally used for preparation of w/o or o/w type of ointments and creams.

Some of the examples of Emulsifiers

Natural	Inorganic	Semi synthetic	Synthetic
Acacia agar tragacanth pectin wool fat chondrus egg yolk, etc.	Milk of magnesia, Magnesium oxide Magnesium tri-silicate Magnesium aluminium silicate	Methyl cellulose Sodium carboxyl methyl cellulose and etc	ANIONIC : Alkali soap, Alkyl sulfates, Lactylates, Sulfosuccinates, Silicones, Taurates, Phosphate ester. NONIONIC : Polyoxyethylene alkyl-aryl ethers, Polyoxyethylene sorbitan esters, Polyoxyethylene fatty acid ester, Sorbitan fatty acid esters, Glyceryl fatty acid esters CATIONIC : Quaternary ammonium compounds, Alkoxyalkyl-amines

Fig. 1.3 Examples of Emulsifiers

6. **HUMECTANT :**

A humectant is a hygroscopic substance . Humectants are used to increase the solubility of the active ingredient, to increase its skin penetration, and to increase the hydration of the skin .

Example of commonly used humectants are Poly Ethylene Glycol, Glycerol or Sorbitol .

7. **BUFFERS :**

In drug formulation pH is important as it affects drug stability, solubility, absorption etc. Buffer resist the changes in pH in normal storage conditions and use. Buffers are added to enhance compatibility with skin , drug solubility, and drug stability

Examples of buffers are sodium acetate, sodium citrate, potassium metaphosphate .

8. **ORGANOLEPTIC AGENTS :**

These are the group of agents such as colouring, flavouring and sweetening agents. Suitable colouring agents like amaranth, brilliant blue etc are used. For flavouring agent vanilla, stawberry, raspberry etc are used to improve the taste of the drug. For sweetening agents like glucose, sorbitol, saccharin etc are used to inprove the palatability and acceptability of a drug.

9. **PRESERVATIVES :**

Preservatives are added to inhibit the growth of contamination of microorganisms and extends the shelf life. e.g. Para-hydroxybenzoate (parabens), phenols, benzoic acid, sorbic acid, etc.

10. **GELLING AGENTS :**

Gelling agents are substance that enhance the thickness or viscosity of the the formulation . It is used to stabilize the formulation. Gelling agents are hydrocolloids or hydrophilic inorganic substances.

Some examples of gelling agents :

Natural	Inorganic	Semi synthetic	Synthetic
Proteins : Collagen Geletain Polysaccharides : Agar Gum Tragacanth Pectin	Aluminium hydroxide Bentonite	Carboxymethyl cellulose (CMC) Methylcellulose (MC) Hydroxypropyl cellulose (HPC) Hydroxyethyl cellulose (HEC).	Carbomer carbopol 940 Carbopol 934 Poloxamer Polyacrylamide. Polyvinyl alcohol Polyethylene.

Fig . 1.4 Examples of Gelling Agents

11. FRAGRANCES :

Fragrances are used in formulation to mask the unpleasant odour of ingredients. Selection of fragrances or right odour is little difficult task.

Examples : rose oil, almond oil, lavender oil and etc .

EVALUATION OF SEMI SOLID DOSAGES FORMS

Semisolid dosage forms are evaluated for different pharmacopeial and non-pharmacopeial tests to determine their physical and chemical, microbial, in- vivo, and in-vitro properties. These evaluation or tests assist in retaining their quality and minimize the variations in batch-to-batch. These are some test for evaluation of semisolid dosage forms:

1. **Homogeneity and Surface Morphology:** The homogeneity of semisolid is commonly evaluated via the surface morphology and visual inspection of gel by means of the use of scanning electron microscopy.
2. **Minimum fill test:** This test is done to compare the labelled weight or volume with weight or volume of product filled into each container. It aids in assessing the product's content uniformity. Only containers containing preparation in amounts no larger than 150 g or mL are subject to a minimal-fill test.

There are two steps to it:

First, labels on the product containers were taken off. Then, weigh them after washing and drying the surface (W2).

Secondly, remove the complete product from every container. Then after cleaning and drying, record the weight of empty containers (W_2). The weight of product = the difference between total weight (W1) and empty container weight (W2).

According to the USP the average net content of 10 containers have to not be less than the labeled amount. If the weight of the product is between 60 and 150 g or ml - then the net content of any container shouldn't be less than 95% of the labeled amount. The product weight is < 60g or mL – then the net content of any container should not be much less than 90% of the labeled amount. If those limits doesn't match then test has to be repeated with an additional 20 containers.

3. **Water Content:** The presence water might affect the microbial, physical, and chemical stability of creams and ointments. For determion of water content in the preparations " Titrimetric method " is normally perform. For determination, special titration setups and reagents - Karl Fischer are used .
4. **pH:** A pH meter is used to determine the pH.One gram of the semisolid formulation (gel) is diluted in 100 mL of distilled water and let to remain for two hours in the pH meter.To maintain the consistent quality, pH dimension is essential.
5. **Leakage Test:** Required for ophthalmic ointments, this test determines whether the ointment tube and its seal are intact. The outer surfaces of ten sealed containers are chosen, and they are cleaned. They are kept at 60 3°C for 8 hours while lying horizontally on absorbent blotting paper. If no tube is seen to be leaking during the test, it is successful. The test is repeated with an additional 20 tubes if leakage is found. If out of 30 tubes, no more than 1 exhibits leakage, the test is considered successful.
6. **Microbial screening:** Microbial contamination of semisolid preparations is not acceptable. As a result, the majority of topical semisolid formulations are checked for the presence of Pseudomonas aeruginosa and Staphylococcus aureus. The USP regularly advises screening for Escherichia coli, Salmonella species, and total aerobic microbial counts. Moreover, yeasts and moulds are checked in formulations intended for rectal, vaginal, and urethral treatments. The existence of microorganisms is screened for using appropriate official microbiological procedures. To estimate the total aerobic microbial counts, the plate method or multiple-tube method is used.
7. **Drug content/Assay:** Several techniques are used to assess the amount of drug contained in a unit weight or volume of a semisolid dosage form. There are chromatographic, spectrophotometric, titrimetric, and frequently microbiological assays carried out. The type of the medicine, its concentration in the product, interactions between the drug and other formulation components, and legal restrictions all play a role in the method's choice.
8. **Extrudability :**. To determine the force necessary to extrude the material from the tube, an empirical test is commonly used. Using an extrudability device, the mass in grammes needed to extrude a 0.5 cm ribbon of gel in 10 seconds is used to calculate the formulation's extrudability.
9. **Studies on stability:** Semisolid dosage forms are subjected to stability tests in accordance with ICH guidelines. The appropriate temperature and relative humidity are applied to the preparations in accordance with the rules, and after a predetermined amount of time, they are checked for various quality characteristics.
10. **Skin irritation and sensitivity study :** No semisolid formulation should have an irritating impact on the skin, mucous membranes, or eyes. The skin and eyes of rabbits or the skin of rats might be used for the irritancy tests. At intervals of 24, 48, 72, and 96 hours, reactions are recorded.Eye irritation is assessed using lesions on the cornea, iris, and conjunctiva. Skin irritation is assessed by the presence of patches on the skin within two weeks.

MODEL QUESTIONS :

1. **Define semisolid dosage forms.**

2. **Discuss all the classification of semisolid dosage forms.**
3. **What are the factors affecting the dermal penetration of drug?**
4. **Discuss the mechanism of dermal penetration of drug.**
5. **Discuss various excipients used in semisolid dosage form.**
6. **Write brief note on :**

i. **Ointments**
ii. **Creams**
iii. **Pastes**
iv. **Gels**

Printed by Libri Plureos GmbH in Hamburg,
Germany